Cosmo's Bedside Quiz Book

27 Great Sex & Relationship Quizzes

D0839316

Cosmo's Bedside Quiz Book

27 Great Sex & Relationship Quizzes

The Editors of COSMOPOLITAN

HEARST BOOKS
A division of Sterling Publishing Co., Inc.

New York / London
www.sterlingpublishing.com

10 9 8 7 6 5 4 3 2

Cover design by Peter Perron
Book design by Judith Stagnitto Abbate
Published by Hearst Books,
A division of Sterling Publishing Co., Inc.
387 Park Avenue South, New York, NY 10016

For information about custom editions, special sales, premium and
corporate purchases, please contact Sterling Special Sales
Department at 800-805-5489 or
specialsales@sterlingpublishing.com.

Manufactured in the United States of America

ISBN: 978-1-58816-487-2

Contents

Contents

Introduction

You picked up this book because you wanted to find out if (a) you deserve the gold in the bedroom Olympics; (b) your Prince Charming is really a frog; (c) your closest pals are *Friends* friends or total back-stabbers; or (d) you're living up to your fun, fearless female potential. If you checked any of these choices then you've come to the right place. The *Cosmopolitan Bedside Quiz Book* is chock-full of info and advice about love, lust, and life.

In the Love arena, you can peer into the future of your relationship with the "Are You a Together-Forever Couple?" quiz. Or scrutinize your new man's character with "Is He Worthy of Your Love?" and "Is He a Keeper?" If you've suffered a series of loser liaisons and are beginning to suspect that *you* might be partly to blame, "Do You Sabotage Your Relationships Without Realizing It?" could help set you straight and lead you to a perfect partnership.

On the ever-important subject of Lust, these quizzes come complete with killer tactics for boosting your sexual self-knowledge and skills. "How Good Is Your Sexual Etiquette?" contains crucial info on handling social interactions most definitely *not* covered by Emily Post. Ever wonder how partners rate your bedroom potential? Check out "What Kind of Sexual Vibe Do You Give Off?" And if you're constantly pestered by icky propositions and men with wandering hands, "Are You a Tease?" may just tell you why.

Men aren't always our primary interest, of course, and that's why the Life section contains a whole series of quizzes all about you. Are you a Giver or a Grabber? A Trauma Queen? A Control Freak? The appropriate *Cosmo* quiz will provide the answer to any one of these questions. Take the quiz "What's Your True Calling?" and formulate a plan to take you from dead-end drone to dream job diva. Depending on your score for "Are You Psychic?" you might discover you've got the answers to all life's questions already and just didn't know it!

So sharpen some pencils and get psyched for self-analysis. (No permanent markers, please, because you may want to redo these someday.) I hope these new and classic *Cosmo* quizzes provide you with all the fun and 411 that they've brought to me and to our millions of readers.

Kate White
Editor in Chief, *Cosmopolitan*

LOVE

Are You a
Commitment-Phobe?

Does the thought of hooking up make you want to hightail? Check out *Cosmo*'s quiz to see if you're set to make love or make tracks.

1. **After the first date, your man leaves a message the next day telling you what a great time he had. You:**
   a. Assume the worst. It's obvious that this one wants you hitched up and shooting out babies by your next date.
   b. Are flattered. It's refreshing to see he doesn't need to play hard to get.
   c. Give him another chance—even though he obviously has desperado written all over him.

2. **You go out to lunch with a friend. After reading the menu you:**
   a. Are overwhelmed by the choices. *You want the turkey club, then again, what if you get it and the pasta is better?*
   b. Ask the waiter to choose something for you. You couldn't live with yourself if your choice sucked.
   c. Get the special. You're always up for a little adventure. Besides it *is* just food.

3. **Your boyfriend asks you to go for a romantic retreat this weekend. You:**
   a. Refuse. What if something better comes up?
   b. Agree, but keep an excuse on hand just in case you have to bail.
   c. Pack your bags. You're overdue for some body-banging fun.

4. **When it comes to the topic of marriage you:**
   a. Scoff at the mere suggestion. No man's going to put you in a headlock of matrimony.
   b. Think about it now and then. Besides, a vibrator can't mow a lawn.
   c. Are receptive—once you find the right guy.

3

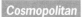

5. **While rummaging through the sale racks you find *the* dress. The store specifies "no returns." You:**
   a. Quiz the clerk, mall security, passersby on the street, and anyone else on whether or not you should go for it.
   b. Leave it on the rack. You might hate it once you get home.
   c. Snap it up. You know a good find when you see it.

6. **For your anniversary, your boyfriend buys you both matching sweaters. You:**
   a. Panic. What's next? Riding around town on a tandem bike?
   b. Gush with excitement, then conveniently lose it—and him—at a later date.
   c. Silently cringe, but graciously accept his argyled attempt at affection.

7. **After an overnight session at your house, you notice your boyfriend leaves his toothbrush at your house. You:**
   a. Clean your grout with it. That'll teach him to fence you in.
   b. Let him keep it there. After all, you don't want him to end up looking like Austin Powers.
   c. On your next date, you return it to him.

8. **Your new man takes you out with his friends and introduces you as his girlfriend. You:**
   a. Are furious. Why doesn't he just lift his leg and urinate on you?
   b. Are a bit surprised, but flattered nonetheless.
   c. Let it slide this time. Besides, it could have been worse. He could have called you his "woman."

9. **Your parents keep needling you about when you're finally going to settle down. Your response?**
   a. "Never. Why have the same thing for breakfast every day when you can have the variety pack?"
   b. "Whenever the timing's right."
   c. "If I get knocked up . . . maybe."

10. **For Christmas, your boyfriend's parents get you a coffeemaker. You:**
    a. Fume. *So that's what they see—a filter-changing housewench ready to serve her man!*
    b. Accept their futile attempt to domesticate you—and hope you don't conveniently mistake Drano for coffee crystals in the future.
    c. Thank them. It could have been socks.

Scoring

1. a–2   b–0   c–1
2. a–1   b–2   c–0
3. a–2   b–1   c–0
4. a–2   b–1   c–0
5. a–1   b–2   c–0
6. a–2   b–1   c–0
7. a–2   b–0   c–1
8. a–2   b–0   c–1
9. a–2   b–0   c–1
10. a–2   b–1   c–0

16 points or more: Track-Making Mama

You'd rather get a prescription filled by Jack Kevorkian than put down relationship roots. Skittish at even the slightest overtures of obligation, you equate settling down with being shackled down, thus leaving you on the lam from long-term love. Your "Escape from Alcatraz" attitude can even bleed over into your everyday decisions. But it's your one-on-one relationships that suffer from your self-governing gumption. "You may have had a mother with a subservient nature, which led to disastrous results," says Guy Corneau, psychologist and author of *Lessons in Love: The Trans-formation of the Soul Through Intimacy* (Holt). "You've become so autonomous that you can't share your life without feeling a threat toward your independent spirit." How do you break free from your lone wolf instincts and catch up with the pack? "You may want to seek therapy to help you figure out why you run from relation-ships," says Corneau. "Or, try to step outside yourself and observe your own actions." The first step is finding out what's behind your "born free" mentality. "Promise yourself that you will take things one step at a time," says Mira Kirshenbaum, author of *Our Love Is Too Good to Feel So Bad: The 10 Prescriptions to Heal Your Relationship* (Avon Books). Once you get a handle on your "party of one" persona, you'll be able to cut those commitment killers off at the pass, and be that much closer to setting a table for two.

8 to 15 points: Borderline Bolter

Although not nearly as phobic as the track-happy chick, you've been known to pull a Houdini now and then when things get heavy. You see commitment as a threat rather than the next step in a blossoming relationship, leaving you to question the intentions of any man who wants to go beyond your first name. "You may have had a bad experience in the past that soured you on settling down," says Corneau. But that doesn't mean you have to be single forever. "Stop making yourself feel as if you're under the gun," says Kirshenbaum. "Let others get panicked—you take all the time you need to get the right fit." The key to halting those hit-the-trail tendencies is to learn that sharing your life doesn't necessarily mean losing it. In fact, strong individualism will make you even more magnetic to your man of the moment.

7 points or fewer: Commitment Cool Chick

You're not one to shy away from a good thing. Rather than running scared from Mr. Right you view commitment as a coup, all the while knowing when to set up camp—and when to pack it in. "You probably had a very trusting relationship with parents who nurtured your independence and self-expression with love and support," says Corneau. As a result, you don't feel the need to run to show that you are your own woman. You know you can trust in yourself to make the best decisions for your life so you're free to love without the flight factor. Just be sure to keep that trailblazing in check and you'll likely never risk choking on your own dust. ✳

Are You a Together-
Forever Couple?

Are you a meant-to-be or a meant-to-flee? Check out *Cosmo*'s quiz to gauge your relationship's shelf life.

1. **You invite him to your best friend's wedding. He:**
   a. Not only helps buy the gift but uses the word "registry."
   b. Agrees, but spends most of the time annoying the bridal party.
   c. Agrees, but spends most of the time *doing* the bridal party.

2. **The night the two of you have front row tickets to a concert you come down with the flu. He:**
   a. Drops off some chicken soup, then takes his sister to the show.
   b. Says, "Hope I don't catch it," then leaves you stranded with a humidifier.
   c. Gives the tickets to a friend and comes to your place to play nursemaid.

3. **Your 12-year-old cat Lewis dies. Your man:**
   a. Waits a few weeks, then takes you to the pound to find a replacement.
   b. Brings you flowers and a framed picture of Lewis.
   c. Presents you with the lovely wrap he had made out of his carcass.

4. **An old boyfriend shows up unexpectedly on your doorstep. Your man:**
   a. Invites him in.
   b. Puts him in a headlock.
   c. Leaves the two of you alone for a long-awaited reunion.

5. **It's been days since he's called. You:**
   a. Stalk the bastard. He should know better than to play with your emotions.
   b. Call when you know he's not home and leave a message on his machine.
   c. Call him and invite him to dinner—you're not one to play waiting games.

6. At a party, a friend holds up a camera, points it at the two of you, and says, "Cheese." He:
    a. Snuggles close and smiles.
    b. Awkwardly puts his arm around your neck and grins.
    c. Says, "Uh, excuse me, honey—you're in the way."

7. While he's away on a business trip you:
    a. Get a good-night call every night.
    b. Never hear from him.
    c. Find a message from him on your answering machine that says "I miss you."

8. His love notes generally commence with:
    a. "Hey Mama"
    b. "My darling"
    c. "Insert name here"

9. During a heated sex session, you blurt out, "I love you!" He:
    a. Covers your head with a pillow and keeps going.
    b. Replies, "That's nice."
    c. Says, "I love you too."

10. Your parents are in town and you invite him to join the three of you for dinner. He:
    a. Says, "Why go out?" and makes his famous lasagne for everybody.
    b. Says he can't make it but shows up for dessert.
    c. Remembers that he has to leave town.

11. While the two of you are taking a walk in the park you pass a couple strolling with their new baby. He:
    a. Says, "You're on the Pill, right?"
    b. Says nothing but takes your hand and holds on tight.
    c. Takes a glance but is quickly distracted by the "bottles" on the breast-feeding mother.

12. His pet name for you is:
    a. "Sweetheart"
    b. "Babe"
    c. "Hoochie Mama"

Scoring

1.	a–2	b–1	c–0
2.	a–1	b–0	c–2
3.	a–1	b–2	c–0
4.	a–2	b–1	c–0
5.	a–0	b–1	c–2
6.	a–2	b–1	c–0
7.	a–2	b–0	c–1
8.	a–1	b–2	c–0
9.	a–0	b–1	c–2
10.	a–2	b–1	c–0
11.	a–0	b–1	c–2
12.	a–2	b–1	c–0

18 points or more: Growing Gray Together

You're the type of couple that makes everyone sick. With your love-bird looks and thumbs-hooked-in-each-other's-pocket strolls, you have obtained what is the Holy Grail of the *Ally McBeal* set: true love. "You've both reached the level where you accept each other as is," say Beatty and Elliot Cohan, authors of *For Better, for Worse, Forever: 10 Steps for Building a Lasting Relationship with the Man You Love* (Chandler House Press), but that doesn't mean you're both blinded by bliss. Quite the contrary: you've learned to love the good, the bad, and the ugly side of your mate, setting the stage for a love built on something more solid than the stuff of grocery store paperbacks. But don't go warp-speed on the wedding plans just yet. "We always advise couples to wait at least six months to a year before making any big decisions," say the Cohans. That way you can be sure that you have more in common than just compatible body parts.

9 to 17 points: Potential Permanency

Don't stock up on the rice just yet. While your relationship has potential to parlay into a permanent pairing, you're not exactly charging toward the chapel. But just because you're not shopping for china patterns doesn't mean you don't have a good thing going. "Love takes time to evolve," say the Cohans. "It's important to learn to be patient and enjoy the process of getting to know one another and allow your love to grow gradually." So how do you know if he's the real thing or a reject? "Look at his willingness to work on the rough spots," say the Cohans. If he's open to discussion about problems and shows a genuine interest in your relationship's well-being, chances are you've scored major mate material. But if he spends most of his time ducking out of discussions, it may be time to bail. "If you think you're going to change him, think again," says Russel Wild, author of *Why Men Marry* (Contemporary Books). Sure anyone can do a tune-up, but if it looks like you're in for a relationship rehaul—best to leave that lemon on the lot.

8 points or fewer: Relationship Rigor Mortis

Sushi has a longer shelf life. Maybe you're in love with the *idea* of love and refuse to acknowledge a losing hand when it's been dealt. The only thing this relationship has going for it is the fact that it's already gone. The question is, Why are you still there? "If he's got fifty percent of what you want," say the Cohans, "that's fifty percent of what you don't want," and all the talking in the world isn't going to tip the odds in your favor. A better solution? Learn from the losing experience and let it lead you to the kind of love you do want. Stop focusing on making it work and instead channel your energy toward making your life better. Once you're the best you can be, real love is bound to find you.✳

Are You Holding Out for a Fantasy Man?
(or, Are You Too Willing to Settle?)

Would you recognize good marriage material if he were right in front of you on bended knee? Take this quiz to see if you're setting your sights ridiculously high . . . or pathetically low.

1. **The dinner check arrives, and your date is short on cash. You:**
   a. Recoil in absolute horror.
   b. Pay for dinner—and the movie.
   c. Pick up the tab, but if he doesn't fork over some moola next time, he's out.

2. **You just found out your new boyfriend has 2 kids from a previous marriage. You:**
   a. Fish around to see if he wants more.
   b. Ask whether he's considered sending them to boarding school.
   c. Spend your free time making fudge.

3. **Your boss just axed you along with your entire department. Your significant other:**
   a. Doesn't return your tearful calls.
   b. Immediately picks you up from the office to commiserate over drinks.
   c. Drops everything to comfort you. Still, you're pissed that he doesn't bring a "recovery vacation" plane ticket.

4. **He kisses like a Labrador: lots of slobber, too much tongue. You:**
   a. Give him a smooching lesson.
   b. Immediately find him a new home.
   c. Overlook it—he has so many other good qualities to concentrate on.

5. **His hair's been thinning the past few months. You:**
   a. Bail. In your book, bald ain't beautiful.
   b. Stick by him. Bruce Willis is way sexier than Fabio any day.
   c. Ignore it—*and* his spare tire.

6. **Your new man goes bonkers every time you get together with any of your male friends. You:**
   a. Think it's sweet. He must really care.
   b. Get an unlisted number right away. What'll be next—stalking?
   c. Sit him down and reassure him that these guys are *just friends.*

7. **He's been spending a lot of time at his high-stress new job. The best way to deal?**
   a. Tell him to take an immediate vacation—or you're history.
   b. Let it slide—he hates it when you nag.
   c. Compromise. You will be more understanding about his long hours if he'll be more responsive at home.

8. **Now that you have been living together a while, you're not having sex so often—though you feel closer to him than ever. Naturally, you:**
   a. Don't panic. Every relationship has dry spells.
   b. Look elsewhere.
   c. Hardly notice. You weren't really that physically attracted to him in the first place.

> A fear of intimacy may be why you set your sights so high.

9. **He tells you he cannot imagine ever settling down with just one woman. You:**
   a. Wait a while to see if he changes his mind. If he doesn't come around relatively soon, you'll make tracks.
   b. Tell him that you're crazy about him, and if you have to share him, so be it.
   c. Figure he's not worth your time. If he were, he'd sacrifice his little black book for you, pronto.

12

10. **On those crucial first few dates, he should be willing to:**
    a. Talk about *anything,* including his most embarrassing moments. How else can you get to know him?
    b. Discuss whatever moves him. And if it's the NBA playoffs, well, you're just happy to have a man who'll talk.
    c. Tell you a bit about his family, his future plans, and hopes. Anything more would be too much too soon.

11. **You were stuck late at work every night last week. Your mate:**
    a. Had you up until midnight cooking dinner—he likes things just so.
    b. Took over all the household duties without your even asking.
    c. Was thoughtless; he didn't iron and made the most uninspiring meals.

12. **Check any of the statements you agree with:**
    a. You'd never date a guy who's not taller than you are—you're allergic to shrimp.
    b. You can tinker with a man, but you can't overhaul him completely.
    c. Every time one of your friends announces her engagement, you panic.
    d. You don't expect your future husband to support you financially.
    e. If sparks don't fly on the first date, you don't accept (or ask for) a second.
    f. You've had lots of brief romances.
    g. You like a guy who's unpredictable.
    h. You drop your friends when you become seriously involved with a man.

Scoring

1. a–3   b–1   c–2
2. a–2   b–3   c–1
3. a–1   b–2   c–3
4. a–2   b–3   c–1
5. a–3   b–2   c–1
6. a–1   b–3   c–2
7. a–3   b–1   c–2
8. a–2   b–3   c–1
9. a–2   b–1   c–3
10. a–3   b–1   c–2
11. a–1   b–2   c–3
12. Give yourself the corresponding number for each item you checked.

a–1   b–2   c–1   d–2
e–3   f–3   g–1   h–1

Now count up the number of 1s, 2s, and 3s you've checked—but don't add them together.

Mostly 1s: Beavis and Butt-head Groupie

So what if he insists on splitting the check at McDonald's? Since you can't imagine doing any better, you don't bother looking for someone who understands the finer points of romance and intimacy. Unconsciously, you may be trying to re-create an unhappy or deprived childhood, says Alan Entin, a psychologist based in Richmond, Virginia. "People who treat you poorly feel comfortable and familiar," he explains. You may also desperately fear getting hurt, adds psychologist Carl Hindy of Nashua, New Hampshire. "You figure you can't be rejected by someone so pathetic."

So, how to stop reeling in bottom-feeders? Ask your friends and family to help by telling you what they *really* think of the unemployed tattoo artist you've been seeing. "Grill them early in the relationship—when they feel they can be honest," advises Hindy. Should that fail, consider therapy as a means of figuring out what fuels your loser lust.

Mostly 2s: The Good-Guy Girl

You don't demand perfection. If he forgets to put the toilet seat back down, that's okay, as long as he meets more fundamental needs. On the other hand, a man who constantly nags you to lose five pounds won't last long with you—which doesn't mean you'll never compromise for him; if he can't stand your wet panty hose all over the apartment, you'll clean up your act. As for sex, you're realistic enough not to ditch him once the initial thrill is gone. "You understand chemistry counts," says Entin, "but also that the key to a long-lasting relationship is friendship."

Mostly 3s: Kennedy Wanna–be

Sorry. JFK, Jr., is taken. But given the chance, you'd probably find plenty wrong with *him*. A fear of intimacy may be why you set your sights too high. "You look for a fatal flaw to avoid engaging in a real relationship," says Entin. Or maybe your self-esteem's so low, you subconsciously figure, "If I'm with *him*, people will think

I'm worth something." In either case, says Entin, a little self-exploration (alone or with a therapist) may help free you from your quest for the ideal man. In the meantime, advises Hindy, if your head says he's a good guy, give your heart a chance to catch up.✳

Is He Worthy of Your **Love?**

Find out whether your man's worthy to worship at the temple of you, is not fit to paint your fingernails, or is just in need of a little TLC (Tender Loving Changing).

1. **You've dressed up for a meeting. His reaction when he sees you:**
   a. "Hey, can I be around when you take those clothes off?"
   b. He doesn't say anything.
   c. "You look nice today."

2. **The boss came down really hard on you at work. Shaken, you feel like crawling into bed and staying there for a week. You call your honey to weep and whine. He:**
   a. Listens, then offers to come over and snuggle. Brings a pint of vanilla swirl.
   b. Cuts the conversation short—he's meeting the guys for beers.
   c. Listens, suggests you get a good night's sleep, and calls the next day.

3. **He makes sure you climax:**
   a. When he does or soon thereafter.
   b. Before he does.
   c. You're on your own, kid.

4. **Out of nowhere, you start getting anxiety attacks. Your boyfriend:**
   a. Helps you hunt down a therapist.
   b. Tells you it's all in your head.
   c. Shows concern but seems a little freaked by your behavior.

5. **You're out to dinner, and when the check arrives, your boyfriend:**
   a. Lets you know your portion of the bill, pointing out that you ordered 2 glasses of wine plus an appetizer salad while he only had a beer and burger.
   b. Says, "It would be my pleasure" when you reach for your wallet.
   c. Puts down cash for half the amount.

6. **When a gorgeous woman walks by both of you, he usually:**
   a. Sneaks a sideways look at her.
   b. Stares at her long and hard.
   c. Says, "Don't worry, darling, she's not even fit to polish your pumps!"

7. **When you both have a fight, you end up feeling:**
   a. Frustrated. He shuts down.
   b. As if you are in the process of working something out. He may get mad, but he always remains rational.
   c. Frightened by his behavior.

8. **You tell your boyfriend that your mom [sister/girlfriend] has just advised you against taking that fabulous new job. His response:**
   a. "Don't listen to her, you'll be great."
   b. "She's just afraid for you. You'll be great."
   c. "I never really liked your mom."

9. **You had a terrific time at the party—sure, you flirted with a couple of men, but it was all in good fun. The next day, your boyfriend would most likely:**
   a. Be turned on by your popularity.
   b. Amorously tell you how lucky he is to be the one who goes home with you.
   c. Sulk and make a snide comment about your drinking.

10. **When both of you spend a weekend together:**
    a. You often feel lonely; he sits in front of the TV a lot, tinkers in the garage.
    b. You're completely comfortable—you both laugh, relax, make love.
    c. The sex is fabulous, though he's lazy about making out-of-bed plans.

11. **How do your friends describe the man you are dating?**
    a. The catch of the year.
    b. A nice man who seems to adore you.
    c. Someone to have fun with but not someone you want to get serious with.

12. **Check any of the following statements that apply:**
    a. When he knows something (a fact or current event) you don't know, he never patronizes you.
    b. He would get allergy shots so he could live with you and your 2 cats.
    c. He's tried to turn you on to whatever sport he's into (golf, kayaking, baseball).

d. You frequently hear from friends that he's been bragging about you.

e. He truly doesn't even notice when you've put on an extra 5 pounds.

f. He brings home unexpected treats for you—CDs of groups you've said you like, articles he's cut out that would interest you, your favorite bakery cookies.

g. He doesn't freak when you cry or accuse you of having PMS.

h. He holds hands and hugs a lot—always makes you feel cherished.

i. If he found a wallet full of money, he'd hunt down the owner and give it back with all the dough.

j. You are comfortable with the amount of alcohol that he drinks.

Scoring

1. a–3   b–1   c–2
2. a–3   b–1   c–2
3. a–2   b–3   c–1
4. a–3   b–1   c–2
5. a–1   b–3   c–2
6. a–2   b–1   c–3
7. a–2   b–3   c–1
8. a–2   b–3   c–1
9. a–2   b–3   c–1
10. a–1   b–3   c–2
11. a–3   b–2   c–1
12. Give yourself 3 points for each statement checked.

More than 44 points: Worthy

"A worthy man is one who makes you feel good when you are around him," says psychologist Michele Kasson, coauthor of *The Men Out There* (Rutledge Books). "The two of you have shared goals and common interests, and you each give the other support in facing the tough, cruel world." He's kind, compassionate, supportive . . . but not just to you. "If he treats his mom—and even the waiter—well," adds Kasson, "then he will be respectful of you too." Remember, though, true love doesn't mean conflict-free love. How do you handle the situation when problems arise? "Do you feel more connected and like you know each other better after a disagreement?" asks Daphne Rose Kingma, author of *Coming Apart* (Conari Press). "Couples who are not threatened by differences but instead see them as a process of discovery have wonderful relationships."

26 to 44 points: Workable

Every man has his good points . . . and his flaws. The question is, Can you live with this man's imperfections—can you even get him to change some annoying behaviors? "We all have a bottom line when it comes to choosing another human being to love," says Kingma. "A woman needs to ask herself, 'Does this man have the one quality that is most important to me in a mate?' It may be that he shares your spiritual values or is willing to communicate. This is the grounding bond that, over time, allows the various imperfections of your relationship to recede."

In addition, we all have a number of things we'd prefer to have in a relationship. Kingma suggests you make a list of 10 characteristics that you would like your man to have. If he has 5, it's probably worth sticking around.

The Moment I Knew He Wasn't Worthy

"He bought the papers on a Sunday morning and then said, 'Can I have $3.50, because I won't have time to read them.' I knew he was cheap, but that was the final straw."
—Suzanne, 31, physical therapist

"He asked me not to tell his ultraconservative friends that I volunteer at Planned Parenthood."
—Linda, 28, magazine writer

"He didn't understand why my sister was angry that her husband went golfing the day she delivered their baby."
—Valerie, 28, book publicist

"My father died, and my boyfriend told me he was 'sorry but couldn't handle it' and promptly disappeared for the next few weeks."
—Tina, 29, music agent

"Also, see how he responds to the fact that he has attributes you dislike," adds Kingma. "He may be a football fanatic; perhaps you can convince him to watch at a pal's house so you can have the place to yourself." Also, remember what's truly important to you. "Forgetting the anniversary of your first date is chump change," says Sharyn Wolf, author of *How to Stay Lovers for Life* (Dutton). "You want to be with the guy who'll sit with you in the doctor's office if you find a lump in your breast."

If there is some aspect of his behavior that you truly can't put up with, then approach changing him in a positive way. "You can only change a man who wants to change," says Kingma. "But he has to be inspired by love, not nagging. If you're a health nut and he expresses a desire to get in shape, you can be supportive, but if six months pass and it hasn't happened, then you've got to decide

10 Signs He's the One

1. He looks at Pamela Anderson centerfolds and insists he doesn't know what the big deal is.
2. He spends the weekend with your family and still wants to date you.
3. On Super Bowl Sunday, he offers to spend the day in bed, painting your toenails and giving you backrubs.
4. He doesn't fall asleep immediately after sex.
5. He lets you use his toothbrush when you crash at his place.
6. He leaves you cute, little "shmoopie" messages every day at work . . . and has for the past 2 years.
7. Even after seeing you in a mud mask, stuffing your face with Ben & Jerry's, he still looks at you the same way he did the moment he first saw you.
8. When you argue with him, he never chalks it up to your PMS.
9. He brings you daisies just because it's Tuesday.
10. He insists on waking up at 5 A.M. just to take you to the airport.

whether or not you can live with this in the long run."

Fewer than 26 points: Worthless
This man dismisses your feelings, has more fun channel-surfing than talking with you, and ogles other women right in front of you. Are you so eager to be with a man—any man—that you will settle for someone so undeserving of your love? "You simply can't be with someone who has more emotional power in the relationship than you do," says Kasson. "If you feel you can't stand up for yourself, then this isn't the right man for you."

Perhaps you're aware that you're stuck in an unhealthy relationship—why is it so hard for you to leave? "Because we all want to be loved and we're afraid no one else will come along again," says Kingma. "But the truth is, every person I've ever counseled who's ended a relationship has found someone better." If you know you need to leave and you can't do it on your own, get some help from trusted friends or even a professional counselor.✳

Do You Sabotage Your Relationships Without **Realizing It ?**

Do you rub out romances with bitching and bullying . . . or suffocate them to death with your nonstop neediness? Take this quiz and learn how to squash the "killer" instincts that leave your relationships DOA. Surprise: you might discover you already have the stuff to keep love alive.

1. **When your current boyfriend asks you about your exes, you answer that:**
   a. You thought you'd found the right guy a few times, but each one broke your heart.
   b. Things didn't work out romantically, but you always ended up really good friends.
   c. If there's justice, they'll face endless tax audits, parking tickets, and root canals.

2. **Your man gets fired by his nightmare of a boss. Automatically, you:**
   a. Insist that he move right in with you; he needs all the coddling he can get.
   b. Tell him he had better land a job before your big romantic getaway—you're certainly not picking up the hotel bill.
   c. Take him to dinner, let him know you're there to help him rewrite his résumé and provide any useful contacts.

3. **You're in bed with him, but the way he's touching you reminds you of your gynecologist—and not in a good sense. Your immediate move:**
   a. Lie still. Only a total bitch would bust him on his sexual technique.
   b. Gently move his hand to a hotter spot.
   c. Tell him you're way too stressed-out for sex, then click on the television set.

4. You both are on your way to a restaurant—the one he always gets lost trying to find. What do you say?

    a. "I always get confused around here. It's a left turn up ahead, right?"

    b. "Can we *try* to remember to make a left turn this time, Columbus?"

    c. Nothing until it's too late. Naturally, you then take all the blame.

5. On your birthday your beau, who is on a tight budget, presents you with a home-cooked dinner and a sappy love song he wrote for you. Your reaction?

    a. "Honey, I wouldn't trade you for Donald Trump in a million years."

    b. "You shouldn't have gone to all that trouble. I could have cooked."

    c. "So, did you *get* me anything?"

6. After a toe-curling session of sex, you're up for pillow talk, but he's down for the count. You:

    a. Snuggle up to him—even after he squirms to the other side of the bed.

    b. Elbow him awake and tell him postcoital cuddling is your god-given *right*.

    c. Tell him the next morning that you'd like a little loving the coming weekend, when his libido won't be all that's "up."

7. After moving in with him, you discover both of you now own twice as much stuff as you need. What to do?

    a. Turn the move into an episode of *Let's Make a Deal*: You'll ditch a chair if he'll sacrifice his plastic dishes.

    b. Insist he donate his furniture to Goodwill. After all, your things *are* better.

    c. Offer to dump all your stuff. You know he'll pay you back—somehow.

8. On the night of your dinner party, he tells you his dad is scheduled for emergency gall-bladder surgery—the next morning. How do you deal?

    a. Tell him the surgery is not until tomorrow; if he can't make it, he's history.

    b. Suggest he stop by for dessert—if he's not feeling way too stressed.

    c. Cancel the dinner. Your friends will understand; he very well might not.

9. For the third night this week, you're working late on a big proposal. Your beau's complaining because he craves more time with you. You say:

    a. "I'm sorry, hon, but I have to get this done. Let's make a date for the weekend."

    b. "How dare you whine at me—I thought I could count on you for a *little* support."

    c. "You're right. My boss hasn't bought my *life*. I'll be home in ten minutes."

10. **He has an annoying habit of picking at his teeth after dinner. You:**
a. Joke that toothbrushes work even better than fingernails.
b. Ignore it. So he's got a few bad habits.
c. Point out his "picking" problem while you're at dinner with friends. That ought to cure him pretty quick.

Scoring

1. a–1 b–2 c–3
2. a–1 b–3 c–2
3. a–1 b–2 c–3
4. a–2 b–3 c–1
5. a–2 b–1 c–3
6. a–1 b–3 c–2
7. a–2 b–3 c–1
8. a–3 b–2 c–1
9. a–2 b–3 c–1
10. a–2 b–1 c–3

25 points or more: Love Crusher

You're a Lee Harvey Oswald of love, rubbing out any potential for romance. Your "passion assassin" tendencies may stem from having been let down previously—either during childhood or in a relationship gone really wrong. You feel that if you don't connive, bully, and manipulate, your needs will never be met, says Susan Jeffers, Ph.D., author of *Opening Our Hearts to Men* (Fawcett). Or perhaps you're simply scared of intimacy, snuffing out a relationship before it has a chance to take hold.

So, how to stop the killer within? For starters, catch yourself every time you express feelings in terms of a put-down or anger, says Carolyn Bushong, author of *The Seven Dumbest Relationship Mistakes Smart People Make* (Villard). "Try 'I'm hurt' or 'I'm disappointed' instead of 'You insensitive lug.' Even 'I'm insulted' will do." Next, give yourself a quota of saying 10 thank-yous to him a day—"even if it's just because he brought you your morning coffee," says Jeffers. Meanwhile, quit your bitching: "If he feels appreciated, he'll be that much more loving."

Ex-Wreckers Confess

Learn from the love mistakes these women made.

- "I used to be a merciless teaser. I knew I'd gone too far when a guy I really liked stormed out on me one night. So I had two choices: either lose my mean streak or lose my man."
- "When it came to fights, I'd bring up some 'crime' a guy had committed two months before. Then I learned to stick to the matter at hand. Now the arguments hardly ever escalate."
- "*Needy* was my middle name; I'd call and pester a guy until he started to let his voice mail pick up. Now when I'm about to say 'I need,' I catch myself and think, *Does this really matter?*"
- "I live with a man but was always coming on to other guys—I just didn't want to miss out on the possibility of something better. Then one day it struck me: I was as bad as all those commitment-phobic men."
- "I was a master put-down artist—until the time he asked me whether he'd gained weight. When I answered that I now knew the difference between dating a babe and 'Babe,' he looked so hurt, *I* started crying."
- "I was the princess of pouting. If he worked late on a Friday night, I'd sulk the rest of the weekend. He finally figured out how to get back at me: ignore me. That took the pout off my pucker."

18 to 24 points: Genius of Love

Nobody's perfect, but when it comes to building a loving relationship, you're pretty darn close. Your secret is deceptively simple: a healthy sense of self-respect. Gently but firmly you show your man that you'll treat him with tenderness and consideration—as long as he returns the favor. "This type knows how to call a guy on his bad behavior without destroying him," says Jeffers.

Also, you're not needy. "You have a purpose in life beyond the relationship," continues Jeffers. "Your friends, your job, your participation in the community are important to you too. If the relationship ended tomorrow, you would hurt, but you know you would survive." Ultimately, it's this love-him-but-*can*-live-without-him outlook that makes men so hot to be with you.

17 points or fewer: Love Fool

You must have the word *doormat* tattooed on your forehead, given the way men walk all over you. The sad thing is, even when he does leave footprints all over your face, you cling even harder—which only drives him further away. Says Jeffers: "Healthy men are terrified of extreme neediness. They know they can't fill the void."

Okay, so how to stop being the girl most likely to get ditched? First, pinpoint those times you feel like you're bending too far backward for a man: "Ask yourself, 'Is this something I want to do—or am I doing it so he'll feel indebted to me?'" says Judith H. Tanenbaum, a Manhattan psychiatrist. You can also make your own demands, adds Dr. Tanenbaum: "If he suggests seeing a guy movie and you're in the mood for a chick flick, say, 'I was looking forward to *My Best Friend's Wedding*—do you mind?'" From there, work up to bigger demands. Last and most important, *don't forget to get a life*, says Gerri Brownstein, a psychotherapist who specializes in couples therapy in Coconut Grove, Florida. After all, only when the relationship stops completely defining your life will you really find the guts to ask for what you want. You'll also stop being the queen of cling. "By developing yourself," explains Jeffers, "you stop being so needy. You become a woman of substance—a woman whom a quality man can really appreciate and love."

10 Signs the Relationship Is Over

1. Over dinner, he excuses himself to go to the bathroom and never comes back.
2. You finally figure out why his roommate doesn't like him bringing anyone over—she's his wife.
3. When you call him the only person you reach is the automated operator telling you the number has been changed to an unlisted one.
4. You read his engagement announcement in the paper . . . and you're not the bride.
5. You're served with a restraining order.
6. While home with the flu, you see him on *Jerry Springer*, revealing his secret crush . . . on your brother.
7. You resort to writing yourself cards and sending yourself flowers on major occasions, just so your friends won't realize he "doesn't believe in material gifts."
8. He e-mails you a note, asking to FedEx him his toothbrush and Dave Matthews CD at your earliest convenience.
9. You spot him on *America's Most Wanted*.
10. After moving in, you realize that he doesn't just love his dog, he *loves* his dog.

Can You Trust Him?

Your man swears he won't sleep around and promises to guard your ATM PIN with his life. This quiz will help you find out whether you should take his word—or just take off.

1. **After a bachelor party, you find a Polaroid of your man with a D-cup stripper on his lap. You ask if any women were there. He replies:**
   a. "Ummmm . . . *no*. It was just us guys guzzling beer and playing poker."
   b. "Well, one woman jumped out of a cake, but I barely noticed her."
   c. "Oh, yeah! You should've seen what Bambi Boom Boom did with a banana."

2. **You ask your man to take care of your canary while you're away. When you come home a week later, he breaks the news: Tweety is taking an eternal dirt nap. What's his excuse?**
   a. "That bird was in sad shape way before I was put in charge. It's not my fault!"
   b. "I raced to the vet when I heard Tweety wheeze—I was too late [*sniff*]."
   c. "I called my sister who is a vet, and she said it didn't sound like a big deal, so I didn't do anything. I'm sorry."

3. **You can't take it! You have to spill your best friend's deepest dirt: she's having a fling with her 17-year-old neighbor. What are the first words out of your man's mouth?**
   a. "Her felony is safe with me."
   b. "You've just made me an accessory to a crime. I'm obligated to turn her in."
   c. "Wait until I tell the guys that Miss Priss is getting bagged by the paperboy!"

4. **You've already worked yourselves into a foreplay frenzy when—oops!—you realize you forgot to buy condoms. His reaction?**
   a. "Don't worry about it. I've got a condom. I'm as careful as you are."
   b. "I won't pressure you to go bareback, even though I *have* tested negative for every STD. I'll run to the drugstore."
   c. "Don't worry, baby. I'll pull out."

5. **He wants to borrow your fresh-off-the-lot convertible to drive to his college homecoming. To prove he's worthy to get behind the wheel, he:**
   a. Offers to take a road test—with you as the instructor. If he fails, no car.
   b. Swears that every single speeding ticket he's ever received has been a cruel O.J.-style mockery of justice.
   c. Tries his hardest to please you in bed, then asks, "Now can I have the car?"

6. **His ex—whom you fondly refer to as "that slut"—calls your man and asks him to dinner. When you tell him you're less than pleased, he:**
   a. Rants about how he's totally over her—yet never says he won't go.
   b. Calls her up right in front of you and tells her it's not a good idea.
   c. Asks you to join them to make sure that nothing of a naked nature goes on.

7. **While making love, you reveal a secret sexual fantasy: being tag-teamed by him and another man. What does he do with this info?**
   a. Nothing. His policy is what goes on inside the bedroom stays in the bedroom.
   b. He gets drunk at a party and makes a lame joke about how your all-time favorite movie is *Threesome*.
   c. He brags to his Neanderthal friend, who in turn informs you that he's "ready for action" whenever you are.

8. **You spot his car at a bar known for its bikini-clad waitresses. He said he'd be watching TV at his buddy's house. Later, you ask how he enjoyed the game. He replies:**
   a. "Bob's TV isn't working, so we ended up going to a total dive bar where we knew the game would be on."
   b. "There's no place better than Bob's! I'll be going over there all season."
   c. "Bob wanted to go to the Bikini Bar, so we did. It was tough keeping my eyes on the screen—but my team won!"

9. **You're having a hair-pulling day at work. You call your man and tell him that you'd be eternally grateful if he would take care of dinner and rent a comedy flick. He:**
   a. Makes pasta and picks up an '80s teen flick—your number one guilty pleasure.
   b. Picks up a pepperoni pizza (his favorite) and *Monty Python and the Holy Grail* (also his favorite).
   c. Leaves a note on the fridge saying: "I'm at Bob's. Don't wait up."

How to Spot a Liar

Have a sinking feeling that your man isn't on the level? Here's how to tell if he's just slinging a load of BS.

His body betrays him. Avoiding physical contact isn't the only clue that his word isn't worth squat. "If he clasps his hands tightly or stuffs them in his pockets, he's really saying: 'I'm keeping something inside,'" explains David Lieberman, Ph.D., a body-language expert. Also, watch out if his hands go up to his face or neck while he's talking, which is an unconscious attempt to distract and hide his lies. Halfhearted gestures—like lazy shrugs and weak smiles—also convey lack of conviction.

He shuts up ASAP. If you suspect he's lying, don't make accusations—just ask innocent-sounding questions. A guilty man will rush to end the conversation. "He knows the longer the interrogation, the greater his chances of getting caught," says Lieberman. Truth-tellers, on the other hand, speak with ease because they have nothing to hide.

He overlooks your lie. Try this sincerity test: when he's in the middle of his spiel, roll in a fib of your own. "When he's telling you about the bar he went to with the guys, mention that you heard there was a fire on that block at the same time," offers Lieberman. If he's bogus, he'll either blow right by your lie or give fake details to corroborate his story. But if he's telling the truth, he'll make a point of saying that he saw nary a fire truck or puff of smoke—just to prove you wrong.

10. You bring him home to meet your parents. The biggest bombshell that he drops over dinner is:
   a. During the drive, you sang along to a Barry Manilow tune on the radio.
   b. You were pulled over for speeding and—unsuccessfully—tried to get out of the ticket by flirting with the policeman.
   c. The last time you brought a guy home, you escaped to a motel for "alone time."

Scoring

1. a–0	b–1	c–2
2. a–0	b–2	c–1
3. a–2	b–1	c–0
4. a–2	b–1	c–0
5. a–2	b–1	c–0
6. a–0	b–2	c–1
7. a–2	b–1	c–0
8. a–1	b–0	c–2
9. a–2	b–1	c–0
10. a–2	b–1	c–0

16 points or more: Honest Beyond Belief

This winner would never intentionally let you down—but if he did, you can be sure he'd be the first to 'fess up about it. "When he makes a promise, he does everything in his power to make it a reality" says Mira Kirshenbaum, couples therapist and author of *Our Love Is Too Good to Feel So Bad* (Avon Books). "And he's mature enough not to put a spin on things."

That said, this nothing-to-hide policy can be a bit unsettling at times.

After all, you don't *really* need to know what Bambi Boom Boom did with that banana, now do you? And if his uncensored honesty is insensitive on a consistent basis, he may be using the truth as an underhanded way to be hurtful. If that's the case, give the candid cad the kiss-off. But if he's just a straight shooter, don't be afraid to let him aim right at your heart.

8 to 15 points: He's Only Human

When he says he's going to do something, you can usually count on it. However, there are situations when his actions don't match his words. "Even good guys go back on their promises to protect their own interests," explains David J. Lieberman, Ph.D., author of *Never Be Lied to Again* (St. Martin's Press). "When he lies about a specific touchy issue, he's doing it because that's what he thinks you want to hear."

Just as long as he never sets out to upset you and keeps confidences when it really counts, this guy is definitely a keeper. And as the relationship deepens, he'll realize he doesn't need white lies to keep love alive.

7 points or fewer: Let-You-Down Loser

Face facts: if your guy has a history of sketchy behavior—he constantly blames others for his screwups and always makes a million empty promises—he's destined to let you down. Even if the guy means no harm, his behavior is bound to put you in a chronic state of frustration and fear. "You will never trust what he says and you won't be able to trust your own judgment about him either," says Kirshenbaum.

Ask yourself *why* you're putting up with the get-set-up-to-be-let-down cycle. You may have bad-boy blinders on—you desperately want the relationship to work, so you overlook all the inconsistencies. "But wishful thinking cannot allow you to lose sight of reality," says Lieberman. So if you're repeatedly slammed by your irresponsible man, move on—or you'll never be able to separate his fiction from fact and get the devotion you totally deserve.✳

Is He a **Keeper?**

Have you ever dated a mediocre man for too long? Or wondered if that decent but sort of obsessive guy will ever mellow out? Take this quiz to see if your boyfriend is a loser—or too good to lose.

1. You're kidding around, and he's making promises you're not sure he can keep. You put your hands over your eyes and ask him to guess what color they are (for those of you in our studio audience, they're green). He says:

a. "They're green. Now will you move your hands so I can kiss you?"

b. "Uh, brown? Blue?"

c. "Most of the time, they're green, like sea glass. But sometimes—like that time we went to the beach and it was really clear and we were near the water—they're blue with golden flecks in them."

2. You lose a bet and take him out for dinner. He:

a. Thanks you a hundred times, says he feels a little weird about letting you pay, and insists on ordering—and paying for—an expensive bottle of wine.

b. Orders the most expensive thing on the menu, commenting that he wouldn't normally get it, but since you're paying. . . .

c. Thanks you, says how nice it is to be taken out, and promises to treat you to dinner next weekend.

3. You and your best girlfriend get in a huge fight right before your third date with him. You're upset and need to talk. He:

a. Tells you he didn't have such a great day either—must be a full moon or something—and asks for a massage.

b. Listens to the story, laughing ruefully and nodding sympathetically at the appropriate times. Then he tells you about a fight he had with his best friend and encourages you to order another drink and dessert since you've had a rough day.

c. Keeps interrupting you to talk about a recent falling out he had with a friend.

When you finally finish your story, he suggests that you and your friend see a counselor, which strikes you as crazy.

4. Your favorite aunt dies and you have to cancel what would have been your seventh date. He:
- a. Sends you a copy of *When Bad Things Happen to Good People* and a mammoth bouquet of yellow roses.
- b. Says "Oh, man, what a bummer" and tells you to call him when you get back from "wherever the funeral is."
- c. Tells you he's sorry and to call him if you want to talk. Then he asks whether you have a ride to the airport, offering to drive you if you don't.

5. You're up most of the night having passionate sex at his place. A little after dawn, you:
- a. Wake up to find him still asleep next to you. When he feels you stir, he grabs you, and the two of you go for another round. Afterward, he smiles and says, "What's for breakfast?"
- b. Are startled awake by him as he stands beside the bed with a tray of eggs Benedict, mimosas, and a rose in a bud vase. "Rise and shine!" he nearly shouts.
- c. Find him at the kitchen table drinking a cup of coffee. "Do you want an Egg McMuffin?" he asks. "There's a Mickey D's across the street."

6. After your first kiss, he looked in your eyes and said:
- a. "Since we met, I've been dreaming about how kissing you would feel, and that was better than anything I imagined. Tell me, how was it for you?"
- b. "You're a great kisser. Will you take off your shirt now?"
- c. "I think you're a great kisser. Let's try that again so I can be sure."

7. You've been together for a month, and one night you decide to bring him to your favorite bar, where a few of your girlfriends are hanging out. He:
- a. Sits next to you with his hand on your leg and doesn't talk much at all.
- b. Talks to your friends, advising them on how to handle their boyfriends. Then he buys everyone a round of drinks.
- c. Smiles and shakes hands with everyone but spends most of the time talking to you. Why should he bother with anyone else when the most beautiful girl in the world is sitting right beside him?

8. **You plan to rent *My Best Friend's Wedding* and head over to his house, but you end up having to work late, so you ask him to pick up the movie. You arrive at his place exhausted and ready to be entertained. He's rented:**
   a. An old war movie, "but it's a really good one—*The Great Escape*."
   b. A three-hour-plus Japanese art flick with subtitles. And dinner will be ready in about an hour—it's a gourmet surprise, but he knows you'll love it.
   c. *My Best Friend's Wedding*. It was all rented out at the video store, so he splurged and bought the cassette. And ordered pizza.

9. **You have sex, and it's passionate and deep and all those things that good sex is supposed to be. In the morning, he professes his desire to get together again soon. You hear from him:**
   a. A couple of days later. He leaves a message saying, "Hey, how are you? Give me a call when you have a minute."
   b. A week later. The message says, "Just calling to see what's up."
   c. Later that day, when his phone call wakes you from a nap. "Hey, it's me. I was just sitting here thinking about you, and I want to see you again tonight. In fact, can I come over in an hour or so?"

10. **He works with a woman who is truly attractive and intelligent. He mentions they had lunch together, and even though you wish you could grin and bear it, you admit you're jealous. He says:**
   a. "What are you worried about? Chicks like that always have boyfriends."
   b. "Yes, I've noticed she's pretty, but she doesn't have anything on you. We should all go out sometime—I think you two would really get along."
   c. "Look, some guys might want to jump on a girl like her, but she's nothing. If it makes you feel any better, I won't talk to her outside of work anymore."

11. **When it comes to sex and especially foreplay, he's:**
   a. Overly enthusiastic. It lasts a long time, and in the middle of everything, he tells you this is only the appetizer—and you can't see how he's still hungry since he's been eating for hours.
   b. Not selfish at all. Sometimes he goes downtown, sometimes he lets his fingers do the walking, and he doesn't hang up until he finds your number.
   c. Clueless. He took you out for dinner—isn't that foreplay?

12. **His last relationship:**
   a. Ended last week, but he swears he's already over her.

b. Was serious. They split up about six months ago, and he's been dating a little.

c. Ended with a fight and her getting out of the car late at night at a busy intersection in a bad neighborhood.

13. In public, he's:

a. Affectionate. He holds your hand at the movies. When you're out to dinner, he brushes your shoulder when he returns to the table from the bathroom.

b. Pretty distant. Sometimes he'll slip an arm around you, like walking from the movie theater to the car, but that's it.

c. A cling-on. He drives with one hand planted on your knee, and when you two are walking he never lets go of your hand or takes his arm from around your waist.

14. You've been going out for about a month when his family comes into town for a week. He:

a. Disappears completely and only calls you after they've been gone a few days—he needed time to recuperate.

b. Is pretty busy while they're around but finds time to have drinks with you a couple of nights and tells you a great story about his father arguing with the Japanese waiter—in Chinese.

c. Takes you to dinner with the family and introduces you as his girlfriend.

15. He's really busy with work and forgets your birthday. When he realizes what he's done, he:

a. Says he's really, really sorry and "I hope you don't think I'm too much of a jerk for forgetting, even though I am." To atone for his sin, he takes you out to dinner and a movie.

b. Has one of those planes that tow advertising banners fly over your house with the message "Forgive me, Birthday Girl!"

c. Says he's not into birthdays.

16. You met New Year's Eve. For your Valentine's Day date, he:

a. Is more than an hour late picking you up and you miss the movie.

b. Cooks you a simple meal and presents you with a card he made himself.

c. Gives you a huge bouquet of flowers and a 10-pound box of chocolates. Dinner is at an overpriced restaurant.

Scoring

	a	b	c
1.	a–2	b–1	c–3
2.	a–3	b–1	c–2
3.	a–1	b–2	c–3
4.	a–3	b–1	c–2
5.	a–2	b–3	c–1
6.	a–3	b–1	c–2
7.	a–1	b–2	c–3
8.	a–1	b–3	c–2
9.	a–2	b–1	c–3
10.	a–1	b–2	c–3
11.	a–3	b–2	c–1
12.	a–3	b–2	c–1
13.	a–2	b–1	c–3
14.	a–1	b–2	c–3
15.	a–2	b–3	c–1
16.	a–1	b–2	c–3

26 points or fewer: Mr. Slacker

If "like" doesn't work for you as an L word, you need to smile and say, "Thank you, good night," to this guy. (And while you're at it, let him pick up the check!) He may be quite friendly, funny, and sexy, but ultimately he's too self-centered to be long-term boyfriend material. Sure, he's up for togetherness if it doesn't require a big investment of time or emotion. But you're not likely to spend hours passionately making out with him or share intense conversations about the significant moments of your respective childhoods. He's just not deep enough for that.

On the other hand, if you're in the mood for something casual, don't pull the plug right away. Provided the guy's at least some fun to be around and he's good in bed (if you're spending time in a relationship that doesn't have legs, you should at least be getting great sex), he might be just the man you're looking for.

In any case, if you find yourself attracted to a man like this, you should ask yourself why. Is it because he's basically unavailable? Are you looking for a project instead of a boyfriend? "A woman may think, *If I can get this distant, inaccessible man to pay attention to me, then I will have really accomplished something,*" says Kathleen

Mojas, Ph.D., a clinical psychologist specializing in relationships. The chances that he'll change, however, "are pretty slim."

Consider yourself warned: Cut your losses and move on or see this guy for who he is and adjust your attitude accordingly.

27 to 42 points: Mr. Keeper

This guy may be "the One." Like your favorite pair of jeans, he's comfortable and hugs you in all the right places. Independent but ready to connect with you, he gives a lot to the relationship without making you feel smothered. He shows plenty of affection but doesn't make you wonder how you suddenly acquired a Siamese twin. He's involved but not obsessive. If you ultimately decide he isn't right for you, he'll be disappointed but not suicidal. In a nutshell, he's your best candidate for a lasting relationship.

Mojas says that when you become involved with a guy like this, you'll sense he's eager to get to know you because he likes you, not because he's desperate to be in a relationship. He's caring and kind but not about to camp out on your front porch so he can see you first thing in the morning.

When you first start seeing Mr. Keeper, you may feel confused at times, like he's sending mixed signals. He seems to like you a lot, but he's not calling you every night or planning dates with you to fill his every free moment. Just keep in mind that he's able to pace himself despite his strong feelings for you because he's self-confident and self-reliant, both admirable qualities in a mate. If he keeps coming back for more but slowly, don't jump to the conclusion that he's not passionate. It's just a matter of style—he's into the slow burn.

This is a guy who has his head screwed on straight, who is self-aware and centered (not self-centered, though), and he's not about to drop everything for the first girl who says yes to dinner. If he doesn't want to give up his Tuesday-night basketball game or skip his night-school French class to take you out, don't feel snubbed. Hey, he won't expect you to give up your life either. Mr. Keeper probably doesn't enter into relationships lightly or without a lot of thought. He doesn't go off like a Fourth of July rocket, all bright glare and flashy colors. He's more like

> # A keeper is like an ocean liner—steady, reliable, powerful, capable of going the distance.

an ocean liner—steady, reliable, powerful, capable of going the distance. Don't climb aboard unless you want to take a nice, long trip with him.

43 points or more: Mr. Maybe

Sometimes you think he comes on too strong; other times you like the attention. He can be a real prince—or a royal pain in the butt. Often hyper and perhaps driven by insecurity, a man like this tends to try too hard to please, especially early in the relationship. Only time will tell whether or not he's a keeper.

Chances are good that he genuinely likes you and wants things to work out in the long run, so he spends a lot of time on the relationship (and if he has it, a lot of money too). The problem is, he can be too intense. You can forget about dinner and a movie—this guy also wants drinks before and after, a long walk in the park, and hey, how about a little post-midnight window-shopping downtown? It's the kind of dating that calls for a long nap afterward.

Instead of letting the relationship take its course, he forces and speeds it along. He invites you to meet his parents before you've even told yours about him. He drops hints about having kids together way too early in the relationship. But while he seems so frantic to please you, he's not really listening to you—much less picking up on your hints that you'd like to take things a little more slowly.

So, why would you become involved? We've all dated our fair share of slackers, so a man who worships us—and tells us how beautiful and special we are—is a welcome change. The question with a guy like this is whether he'll mellow over time. Keep in mind that a guy who errs on the side of putting too much into a relationship may just be inexperienced. But that doesn't mean he isn't a keeper. In fact, he can make a great long-term mate if he eases up a bit. This may happen naturally, after he feels more comfortable with you—and sure of himself and the relationship. Or you may just have to tell him you'd like to slow down.

Obviously you don't want to blow off a great guy who just happens to be supersweet and attentive. So you have to trust your instincts about whether he's really into you—or over-the-edge obsessed. If it's the latter, says Sharyn Hillyer, a Los Angeles marriage and family therapist, "You'll start to feel that there are strings attached. And you'll never be able to satisfy such a person or give enough back." ✳

5 Signs He's in Love with Love ... Instead of You

1. On your first date, he gazes deeply into your eyes and swears he's never felt this way before.
2. On your second date, he tells you he's fallen in love with you.
3. From day one, he calls you at least 5 times a day, "just to hear your voice."
4. From the get-go, he ends each conversation with "I love you, darlin'," but he never calls you by your name.
5. He sends a dozen long-stem red roses to your office every single day, accompanied by notes quoting *Romeo and Juliet.*

What Type of Men
Do You Attract?

There are all types of guys out there and we've split them up into 5 categories. Take this quiz to find out if you attract the wildest or mildest—or if they're somewhere in between.

1. As a rule, the men you date:
   a. Expect you to pick up the tab.
   b. Insist on paying.
   c. Pay the tab, resent it, and use this as a reason to stop seeing you.
   d. Never take you out.
   e. Expect you to pay your share or take turns picking up the tab.

2. The men you see are:
   a. Overly romantic and affectionate.
   b. Affectionate, as long as you do things their way.
   c. Seldom affectionate or are affectionate early in the relationship but less so as time goes on.
   d. Affectionate only in bed, if then.
   e. Affectionate more often than not.

3. When you discuss a problem you're having, a man usually:
   a. Mentions one of his own that is worse than yours.
   b. Tells you how to handle it.
   c. Avoids you.
   d. Assumes that you are strong enough to cope with it alone.
   e. Offers to discuss it with you—and supports your decision.

4. When you meet a man and he says he'll call, he:
   a. Calls the next day and every day thereafter.
   b. Calls but seems too busy to talk.
   c. Doesn't call.
   d. Calls at midnight and asks if he can come over.
   e. Calls when he says he'll call.

5. **When you're with a man and there are other women around, he:**
   a. Is oblivious to them.
   b. Notices them, flirts a little, but tries to protect your feelings.
   c. Flirts incessantly and dashes from woman to woman.
   d. Talks about how attractive the other women are.
   e. Is friendly with them but not disrespectful to you.

6. **After you've had sex, a man often:**
   a. Needs to talk to you or be with you.
   b. Becomes possessive.
   c. Rolls over, goes to sleep, and/or never calls you again.
   d. Forgets your name.
   e. Treats you the same as before.

7. **When you call men you're interested in, they usually:**
   a. Love it and encourage you to call.
   b. Make it clear that *they* are supposed to call *you*.
   c. Act too busy to talk or rush you off the phone.
   d. Say they'll call you right back and don't.
   e. Act the same as when they call you.

8. **In arguments, the men you date:**
   a. Give in and do it your way.
   b. Make you believe their way is right and yours is wrong.
   c. Let you have your way but hold a grudge.
   d. Ignore your point of view.
   e. Negotiate.

9. **When a man you're involved with has a problem, he:**
   a. Talks about it incessantly and wants your advice.
   b. Makes his problem seem insignificant in comparison to yours.
   c. Says, "What problem?"
   d. Pretends it's *your* problem.
   e. Tells you he's upset but lets you know he can handle it himself.

10. **When you cry, the men in your life often:**
    a. Cry too.
    b. Are like putty in your hands and will do anything for you.
    c. Withdraw.
    d. Don't take you seriously.
    e. Understand but aren't manipulated by your tears.

11. When you first meet a man, he:
a. Reveals himself but asks little about you.
b. Wants to know all about you but reveals little of himself.
c. Comes on strong, then peters out after a few dates.
d. Doesn't tell you much about himself or ask much about you.
e. Tells you about himself and wants to know about you.

12. Usually, a man's first priority is:
a. Being in love.
b. Working and making money.
c. His buddies, or exercise and sports.
d. Anything except you.
e. Maintaining a balance between you and his career and other interests.

13. Most men give you:
a. Their emotions but not their money.
b. Their money but not their emotions.
c. Everything, at first, and nothing later.
d. Nothing.
e. Both their money and their emotions, and expect you to do the same.

14. When the men you know become upset or angry, they often:
a. Talk about the problem but do nothing about it.
b. Handle it themselves without letting you know they are upset.
c. Clam up.
d. Blame you for everything.
e. Tell you they're upset, why they are, and what they want.

15. You find most men:
a. Overly emotional.
b. Protective of your feelings but not emotional themselves.
c. Appear to be sensitive but aren't.
d. Cold and insensitive.
e. Emotionally available but not whiny.

16. When you have an opinion, men you know usually:
a. Overvalue it.
b. Have a what-would-you-know-about-that attitude.

c. Seem attentive at the time but later don't remember what you said.
d. Ignore it.
e. Listen carefully, even if they don't necessarily agree.

17. **Men seem to be more interested in you when you:**
   a. Act strong and in control.
   b. Are weak and at their beck and call.
   c. Act disinterested.
   d. Chase them.
   e. Feel happy about yourself.

18. **In arguments, you usually end up:**
   a. Feeling like you've been unnecessarily cruel.
   b. In a power struggle.
   c. Having no one around to argue with because they leave.
   d. Feeling like you've been taken advantage of.
   e. Talking it out and resolving the problem.

19. **When you're upset with a man, he:**
   a. Feels guilty and apologizes, even if it isn't his fault.
   b. Criticizes you or accuses you of overreacting.
   c. Avoids you.
   d. Acts as if nothing is wrong.
   e. Asks you what the problem is.

20. **In relationships, you feel:**
   a. Like you have all the responsibility.
   b. Like he knows more than you.
   c. Like he's searching for your flaws.
   d. Used and abused.
   e. Appreciated.

Add up all a's to see if you attract wimps, b's for daddies, c's for Peter Pans, d's for outlaws, and e's for healthy men. Don't be surprised if you attract different types. Outlaws and Peter Pans, for example, share some similar traits.

WIMPS are the kind of men we attract when we appear to be emotionally and/or financially strong. They're looking for women who can mother or even father them. Sometimes they seem refreshing because they're emotional—but don't let them fool you. They're emotional only about what they need from you, and they can never be there for you.

0 to 3 a's
Although you may control men from time to time, you let few, if any, drain you or leech on to you.

4 to 7 a's
Although you don't let men drain you dry, you need to be more careful about what you do for them.

8 to 13 a's
You tend to become involved with men who rely on your strength. Don't let them take, take, take without giving you something in return.

14 to 20 a's
You are a beacon of strength for wimps and probably attract them in droves. Be careful that they don't drain you of your emotional or financial resources. Try making some demands on them for a change.

DADDIES are the kind of men we attract when we're weak and needy. They're attracted to us because our insecurities make them feel strong. They maintain control by giving us protection, advice, and material things as trade-offs for emotional love. They keep us down by preventing us from trusting ourselves.

0 to 3 b's
Although you like to be taken care of from time to time, you're basically a grown woman and not someone's little girl.

4 to 7 b's
You let men take control more often than you should, but you can stand on your own.

8 to 13 b's
You have a tendency to rely on men instead of yourself. You must develop more self-confidence.

14 to 20 b's
You attract men you want to run your life. You must try to take charge of your own life.

PETER PANS are attracted to us as long as they feel no emotional pressure. When they do, they withdraw. They may be workaholics, sportaholics, or exerciseaholics who escape from emotion in their addictions. They may be dance-away lovers who run at the first sign of imperfection, or sexual con artists who chase sex without responsibility. They love the thrill of the chase, but once the chase is over, they fly away from the emotional responsibility of the relationship.

0 to 3 c's
You may have gone after this type and lost before, but now you probably know a Peter Pan when you see one.

4 to 7 c's
You have a tendency to go after this type, but can probably also let go when you have to.

8 to 13 c's
Getting involved with men who will never be there could be a problem for you.

14 to 20 c's
Look out. You attract men who fear emotional commitment, and you could get hurt.

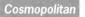

OUTLAWS are attracted to women who demand very little. They're self-involved, self-serving men who give nothing and take everything. They play on a woman's fear of rejection. They come in a variety of types from cowboys to married men. They're disrespectful and gain control by making a woman feel unworthy.

0 to 3 d's
You've met a few, but your self-respect prevents you from getting involved with outlaws.

4 to 7 d's
You let men treat you more disrespectfully than you should because you don't recognize what's happening. But once you do, you get out.

8 to 13 d's
You attract more than your share of outlaws. To salvage your self-esteem, tell them what you won't put up with when you feel you're being taken advantage of. Then go through with it.

14 to 20 d's
Outlaws ride roughshod over you. You must defend your rights and not be ruled by fear of rejection.

HEALTHY MEN are attracted to healthy women who are strong and capable, yet warm and feminine. These men aren't afraid to be emotional and can solve their own problems. They're not afraid of intimacy, although they don't want to be possessed by a woman.

0 to 3 e's
Think about the men you attract, and why healthy men aren't drawn to you. You probably have many unresolved issues about relationships.

4 to 7 e's
You know some healthy men and probably attract some not-so-healthy men too. Work on becoming more secure in yourself, and you'll know as many healthy men as you want.

8 to 13 e's

Many healthy men find you attractive. You, too, must be pretty healthy.

14 to 20 e's

Lucky you. You have a strong sense of yourself, and men know it and respect you for it. ✳

How Deep
Is Your Love?

More than one ingredient goes into creating a *durable* relationship. Does *your* romance have the proper bonding materials?

The Triangular Love Scale

Fill in the blank spaces with the name of the man you love. Then rate your agreement with each of the items by using a 9-point scale in which 1 equals *not at all*, 5 equals *moderately*, and 9 equals *extremely*.

1. I am actively supportive of _____ 's well-being.

2. I have a warm relationship with _____.

3. I am able to count on _____ in times of need.

4. _____ is able to count on me in times of need.

5. I am willing to share myself and my possessions with _____.

6. I receive considerable emotional support from _____.

7. I give considerable emotional support to _____.

8. I communicate well with _____.

9. I value _____ greatly in my life.

10. I feel close to _____.

11. I have a comfortable relationship with _____.

12. I feel that I really understand _____.

13. I feel that _____ really understands me.

14. I feel that I can really trust _____.

15. I share deeply personal information about myself with _____.

16. Just seeing _____ excites me.

17. I find myself thinking about _____ frequently during the day.

18. My relationship with _____ is very romantic.

19. I find _____ to be very personally attractive.

20. I idealize _____.

21. I cannot imagine another person making me as happy as _____ does.

22. I would rather be with _____ than with anyone else.

23. There is nothing more important to me than my relationship with _____.

24. I especially like physical contact with _____.

25. There is something almost "magical" about my relationship with _____.

26. I adore _____.

27. I cannot imagine life without _____.

28. My relationship with _____ is passionate.

29. When I see romantic movies and read romantic books, I think of _____.

30. I fantasize about _____.

31. I know that I care about _____.

32. I am committed to maintaining my relationship with _____.

33. Because of my commitment to _____, I would not let other people come between us.

34. I have confidence in the stability of my relationship with _____.

35. I would not let anything get in the way of my commitment to _____.

36. I expect my love for _____ to last for the rest of my life.

37. I will always feel a strong responsibility for _____.

38. I view my commitment to _____ as a solid one.

39. I cannot imagine ending my relationship with _____.

40. I am certain of my love for _____.

41. I view my relationship with _____ as permanent.

42. I view my relationship with _____ as a good decision.

43. I feel a sense of responsibility toward _____.

44. I plan to continue my relationship with _____.

45. Even when _____ is hard to deal with, I remain committed to our relationship.

Scoring Key for the Triangular Love Scale

Psychologist Robert Sternberg, who developed the Triangular Love Scale, believes there are 3 components to love—passion, intimacy, and commitment—so you will need to tally 3 separate scores for this scale. The first 15 items reflect intimacy, the second 15 measure passion, and the final 15 items reflect commitment. Add your scores for each group of 15 items to find the degree to which you experience these 3 components of love for your partner. You can use the information below to see how you compare with the surveyed group of men and women (average age: 31; either married or in a close relationship).

How Do You Compare?

Score

Intimacy	Passion	Commitment	Percentile
93	73	85	15
102	85	96	30
111	98	108	50
120	110	120	70
129	123	131	85

About Love

Sternberg says that love is like a triangle, and the best kind of love is an equilateral triangle—one in which all three sides are of equal length. What he means, of course, is that love is best when we experience intimacy, passion, and commitment in approximately equal intensities. So you are fortunate indeed if your scores in all three categories were about average and about the same.

If your scores on the 3 dimensions of love are widely different or if you had 1 or 2 scores below average, it does not necessarily mean that your relationship is in trouble. All relationships have their ups and downs, and it is likely that the scores you'd obtain a year from now would be quite different from the scores you have today. You might want to take the test a second time and respond as you would when you are feeling best about your partner. This could give you an indication of the potential of your relationship.

Your scores are also likely to reflect how long you have been with your partner. We tend to become involved in a romantic relationship because we experience the right "chemistry"—or what Sternberg calls "passion." So this component is usually highest during the first year or 2 of a relationship. While passion tends to lose its intensity over time, the most successful relationships continue to maintain a healthy dose of this element.

The second stage of a relationship is generally marked by the development of intimacy. Once we decide we are attracted to a man, we begin to confide in him; we want to share all our secrets with him, to tell our loved one our life story. This component tends to reach its peak a year or 2 after the relationship has begun, but the most successful relationships maintain a high level of intimacy indefinitely.

At some point—maybe after 6 months, maybe 6 years—we develop a sense of commitment to our partner. We value the relationship enough that we will do whatever we can to maintain it. It is this sense of commitment that helps us weather the difficult times that are a part of every relationship. Commitment tends to be strongest for couples who have been together for several years.

The happiest couples are those who have similar love triangles for each other. Sternberg, who obviously remembers his high school geometry well, calls this "congruency." In other words, if you have strong passion for your partner but are a little low on intimacy, you are likely to have problems if your partner is highest on intimacy and lowest on passion. We are happiest in a relationship when our partner feels about us the way we would like him to. You may want the man you love to complete this test so you can determine how compatible the two of you are. It would be nice to discover that you have congruent love triangles. ✳

Cosmo's Ultimate Couple's Quiz: Are You Combatable or **Compatible?**

You like him, but . . . He loves you, but . . . Here's how to forecast if you two will click long-term and eliminate all the agonizing ifs, ands, or buts!

It's been 6 months: the sex is still sensational, the passion still primal. Then, in the heat of tearing off each other's clothes, the truth dawns on you. His boxers, his polo shirt, and his socks will stay where he left them—in the middle of floor. That is, until you pick them up. Suddenly, you begin to notice other little irritations, like the fact that he can't sleep if the temperature is 1 degree above 40, and he has a very short temper. You can't help wondering, *Are the two of you a match made in heaven or is your love going to go to hell?*

"The key to a good relationship lies in being compatible, not just being in love," says C. E. Rollins, author of *Are We Compatible?* (Thomas Nelson). "Compatibility allows relationships not only to function well but to be pleasant, meaningful, and *lasting*." But exactly how *much* compatibility does a couple need to catapult from that first hormonal rush to 'til-death-do-us-part commitment?

"When it comes to what matters most to either of you, you should at least be in the same ballpark," advises Denver-based clinical psychologist Susan Heitler, author of *The Power of Two: Secrets to a Strong & Loving Marriage* (New Harbinger). "It's most important to be matched on the deeper dimensions—your values, religion, whether or not you want to have kids. When there are a lot of differences, there's a lot more to negotiate. And when those differences are about deeply felt issues, it makes negotiating much tougher. In fact, trying too hard to accommodate each other in any of those basic areas is a sign that the relationship is probably not going to work out long-term."

To find out whether your relationship has the feel of custom-made shoes or whether you'll rub each other the wrong way no matter how far you walk together in life, take our ultimate compatibility quiz. Devised to calculate just how well-matched you and your man are, it covers the 6 major aspects of everybody's life: temperament, daily habits, money, sex, work, and values. First, answer each question for yourself, then go back over the quiz and mark—honestly—how you believe your man would respond. If you find points of incompatibility, don't be devastated. "Look, people aren't clones. There are always going to be differences, but some differences are more negotiable than others," explains Heitler.

By taking this quiz, you'll see what's working big-time for the both of you and what you still need to work out. So before you take your current relationship a step further, why not figure out whether or not you can—or should—make the compromises necessary for the relationship to fly?

Your Basic Natures
1. **Your fight style:**
   a. You're a yeller—it's the only way to vent.
   b. You take time out until you're ready to discuss calmly the issue that led to the blowout.
   c. Why fight when most things in life aren't worth it?

2. **Your ideal vacation is:**
   a. Splurge city: sipping umbrella drinks by the 4-star-hotel pool, then dressing up for gourmet dinners.
   b. Nature's way: hiking and biking by day, camping out under the stars at night.
   c. Culture fest: strolling through museums and city streets, bargaining at marketplaces with the locals.

3. **When it comes to catching a flight, you get there:**
   a. 2 hours ahead of time—anything less would leave your stomach churning.
   b. With only 15 minutes to spare—you hate wasting time sitting around in airports.

52

c. 45 minutes early—anything more leaves you feeling angry; anything less, tense.

4. **He's off to Atlantic City with the boys. You feel:**
   a. Mopey. You hate time apart.
   b. Okay. It'll give you a chance to catch up with your own friends. But the next weekend away had better include you.
   c. Thrilled. It's just like being single again.

5. **Check all that apply:**
   a. You're a people person—you can't go to a party without making a new friend.
   b. You mull things over for hours before making any decision.
   c. You blow up easily.
   d. You forgive—and forget—before an apology is even out.
   e. Nothing's sacred to you—you tell your friends *everything*.
   f. You always see life's funny side.

Daily Habits

6. **Your ideal nighttime bedroom temperature is:**
   a. Fit for a polar bear.
   b. As hot as a Caribbean island.
   c. A moderate 68 degrees.

7. **When friends come over to your apartment, they:**
   a. Trip over the laundry and old magazines and newspapers to get to the sofa.
   b. Feel right at home—your place is comfortable and tidy, not intimidating.
   c. Know to take their shoes off before setting one foot on your spot-free carpet.

8. **Your favorite way to fall asleep on a nonsex night is:**
   a. Watching the news.
   b. Reading a good book.
   c. Talking until you drop.

9. **Your feelings on pets?**
   a. Animals are great—when you're watching them on the Discovery Channel.
   b. You can't imagine life without a menagerie that would rival Noah's.
   c. Your one 4-legged friend makes life fun—any more would be a chore.

10. Check all that apply. You:
a. Smoke.
b. Eat vegetarian.
c. Keep abreast of current events.
d. Gossip.
e. Work out regularly.
f. Always need to have the TV or stereo on.

How the Dough Goes

11. When the bills come in at month's end, you:
a. Make minimum payments to keep your credit rating in good standing.
b. Pay off as much as you can without leaving yourself short of fun money.
c. Pay them in full—your rule is never to charge more than you can afford.

12. When it comes to gift giving, you:
a. Love to indulge the ones you love—even if you blow more than you'd planned.
b. Find the perfect (budget-friendly) little something that shows you care.
c. Don't like to dole out too much dough—it's the thought, right?

13. You just got a huge bonus. You:
a. Sock it into your savings plan.
b. Splurge on the vacation of a lifetime.
c. Buy some desperately needed living room furniture and invest the rest.

14. You are out to dinner with a friend. When the tab comes, you:
a. Make sure both of you pay according to what you ate—springing for her six-dollar dessert will only make you stew.
b. Split everything down the middle—why haggle over a couple of bucks?
c. Grab the check—you love to treat people.

15. Check all that apply:
a. You're a big tipper.
b. Ritual splurges (a massage, designer outfit, CDs) save your sanity.
c. You save all year for one vacation.
d. You eat out at least twice a week.
e. You shop at outlets.
f. You buy generic-brand coffee instead of gourmet-brand.

The Sex Connection

16. You best like to have sex:
- a. First thing in the morning.
- b. Right before turning the lights out—better than any sedative.
- c. Any and all times.

17. How often do you need to get it?
- a. 5 to 7 days a week.
- b. Weekends.
- c. Every 10 days would be fine.

18. Your dream sex night includes:
- a. Role-playing, major whipped-cream action, X-rated videos of yourselves.
- b. A warm bath together, candles, and lots of cuddling before and after.
- c. Lingerie and minor-league dirty talk.

19. Location, location, location: Your favorite place to interface is:
- a. In bed, mostly, though you love the occasional session at a semisecluded area.
- b. On an airplane, elevator, sandy beach—you like the risk of maybe getting caught.
- c. In bed—and only in bed.

20. Check all that apply:
- a. You like to talk about sex—i.e., new stuff to try, what turns you on.
- b. A little harmless flirting doesn't bug you.
- c. Making out in public grosses you out.
- d. Giving (and getting) oral sex is a–okay.
- e. Minor kinks (i.e., fur-lined handcuffs, feathers) don't faze you.
- f. You will do it to make the other person happy, even if you aren't in the mood.

Does It Work When It Comes to Work?

21. After a particularly hard day at the office, you:
- a. Talk until you get it out of your system.

> A long-term relationship takes *work*, which means you don't just need sexual fireworks, you need to be able to get along.

55

"When I Knew It Was Over"

Real men and women tell how they knew when the relationship was through.

"My fiancé and I argued about money a lot, but when he joined an expensive gym while we were eating tuna sandwiches, I knew it would never get any better."

—Lisa, 37, public relations exec

"Tina was an utter slob and completely unwilling to change. After a while, it wasn't the mess so much as it was an issue of respect. It was as if every dirty dish was her way of saying, 'You're not worth the compromise.' If she couldn't make the effort on such little things, I wondered what was in store when we faced real issues."

—Tim, 32, professor

"Bob and I met in college, and because I come from a divorced family and have never been close to either of my parents, I always admired Bob's relationship with his family. But after graduation, we moved in together, and the whole family thing got out of hand. He'd call me at work during the week and say he'd be having dinner at his mom's. He'd tell his mom every detail about our lives to the point where I felt my privacy was invaded. In the end, I felt suffocated by how tied he was to his family."

—Terry, 30, banking exec

b. Discuss for a half hour, then put it aside.
c. Check your stress at the front door.

22. When your partner has to put in a 70-hour workweek, you feel:
a. Superneglected—a workaholic isn't what you bargained for.
b. Understanding—a secure future means occasionally logging long hours.
c. Thrilled—a fast-tracker is your fantasy come true.

23. You work to:
a. Make fabulous amounts of money.
b. Fulfill yourself creatively.
c. Pay the bills.

24. If baby were to make 3, you would feel comfortable:
a. Hiring a nanny—both you and your partner want to keep working full-time.
b. Cutting 1 parent's office hours down—work is important but so are the kids.
c. Cutting 1 parent's office hours out—kids need either a mom or a dad at home.

25. You would totally understand (check all that apply):
a. A last-minute business trip.
b. An all-work weekend.
c. Canceling on dinner with Mom and Dad because of a work emergency.
d. Calling the boss from a vacation and begging for 2 extra days.
e. Always being within 500 feet of a fax/modem.
f. Skipping an all-company river-rafting retreat to be with him.

Your Value Systems: Are They in Sync?

26. How much of a role should religion play in your life?

a. A *lot*. You believe strongly in God and are a devout worshiper.

b. A little. You observe the major holidays and occasionally attend services.

c. None. Religion is meaningless to you.

27. You're going to be late with a report because, the truth is, you've been slacking off all week. What do you tell the boss?

a. The truth. You let her know it won't happen again and that you'll work all weekend.

b. That Accounting never gave you all the materials, but being the good sport you are, you'll work all weekend.

c. That your uncle died. You're pretty broken up, would she mind waiting until the middle of the following week?

28. A coworker announces a fund-raising walk for cancer. You:

a. Commit to a twenty-five-dollar donation.

b. Mumble that you already gave cash.

c. Not only sign up but enlist 100 friends to sponsor you, recruit them to walk, and help organize water stations as well.

29. In your opinion, the perfect way to raise kids is:

a. With as many enriching activities as humanly possible—beginning at 9 months.

b. To leave them alone. Your job is to make sure they don't mouth off at the teacher.

c. By letting *their* interests be *your* guide; if they love finger painting, you'll sign them up for art class.

30. Check all that apply:

a. We share the same religion.

b. We grew up living under similar economic circumstances.

c. We come from the same ethnic or cultural background.

d. We have the same level of education.

e. We agree on whether or not to have kids and how many.

f. We have families that are equally functional—or dysfunctional.

Scoring

Now that you've answered this quiz for both yourself and your man, go back and count how many his-and-her responses matched up. Your score will tell just how well-suited you and your suitor are.

40 matches or more: Match Made in Heaven

In the big Peg-Board of life, you've found a natural fit. You both groove on every (or almost every) couple-threatening issue. This level of compatibility is a predictor that your relationship can weather a lifetime of life's little storms. "Through all those frantic, frenzied, and exhausting hours of raising children and dealing with the business of having a life, it's important to know "Can we work together?" says C. E. Rollins. "After all, marriage or a long-term romantic relationship is *work*, which means you don't just need sexual fireworks, *you need to be able to get along.*"

One warning: you may have scored high, but just make sure you racked up all those points in the right places. Questions about bedroom temperature and dinnertime are much more easily negotiated than, say, money matters and sexual styles. "What mainly counts when it comes to compatibility is having similar values and temperament," says Rollins. In other words, your upbringing, your religious beliefs, and your values all contribute to the *basic* person you really are. If you compromise on these core issues, then no matter how well you two may harmonize in other areas, as a couple, you will ultimately clash . . . and burn.

24 to 39 matches: Maybe Match

You may have a problem here if you're looking long-term: it's not just the "toothpaste cap" compromises; your struggles go a little deeper—like whether to raise the kids with religion and how the bucks get budgeted. But don't freak. Even if you and your man aren't carbon copies, "you can bridge relationship gaps through compromise, accommodation, and dedication to working through differences," says Rollins. But that means both of you have to be *committed* to staying together.

For starters, we suggest you go back over the quiz and figure out where the divisions lie. "Then," says Heitler, "ask yourself the following question: Can a deal be cut?" For instance, suppose you like to lounge on vacation, but your man's Mr. *National Geographic* Explorer. Are you willing to negotiate—for instance, head to a spa in South America where you veg out during the day while he climbs through ruins? (Naturally, you will meet up for cocktails at sunset.)

Next, look into your heart and decide whether your differences are really that big a deal. Maybe you're an outgoing butterfly, while he's a shy lone wolf. "An introverted person may be reluctant to attend events with her more gregarious partner, but this can all be negotiated," says Heitler. "What's more important is that the couple enjoy each other's company at *home*. But if your man is *always* silent and you're uncomfortable with that, this may be the type of crack in a relationship that can develop into a very big crevice."

Keep in mind that a little mismatching can be healthy. Say he's a dreamer, while you're grounded in the material world. Believe it or not, the news can be good: after all, someone needs to keep track of paying bills while the other keeps things playful. "Just be sure to keep valuing these differences," says Heitler.

Okay, now that you've figured out what you can live with, it's time to investigate the deal breakers. The biggest stumbling blocks for most couples are money and sex. He's a tightwad while you're the first to shout "Drinks on me!"? "You will need an *exceptionally* strong commitment to talk through this difference and create a spending style with which you're both comfortable," says Heitler. And if you both have drastically different sexual preferences and libidos, all the counseling in the world won't make the kind of match that'll lead to a 5-alarm fire.

Still waffling? Trust your gut. "I counseled a woman who was anxious about her engagement," says Heitler. "The man was terrific. On paper, he seemed perfect. But she felt their souls were too different. In other words, it simply has to *feel* like you belong together. Rational calculating won't get you the whole way. You need to listen to your inner voices."

Ultimately, ask yourself this: 20 years from now, when you wake up next to him, do you picture yourself wanting to start *another* day with him?

Fewer than 24 matches: No Match in Hell

The real question here is, How have you managed to stick it out for so long? If you look back over the quiz with a clear eye, you'll see that your answers reflect very few similarities, therefore very little compatibility. But, you insist, opposites attract. Well, they do for a fleeting, fiery flash, but such couplings usually fizzle fast. "Over time, differing temperament, interests, and points of view tend to gnaw away at attraction," says Rollins.

Still, you love the way he kisses, and you could kiss him for the rest of your life. "But do you like the way he spends the rest of the time when he's not kissing you?" asks Rollins. "That's what's going to matter to you a whole lot more in five years. Most marriages break down because they don't survive the *daily* stuff."

The fact is, staying in a relationship with minimal meshes can lead to big messes. Right now, you're head over heels, but give yourself another nine months, says Rollins, and you'll probably start feeling the turbulence. And don't think you'll be able to change him or even that he'll change himself. "That's not likely to happen," says Rollins. "He is who he is." So if you find that heartache outweighs happiness, you're probably better off making your escape *now*.✳

LUST

How Good Is Your
Sexual Etiquette?

Are you the Queen of Denial—or as venomous as a snake—when something gets messy between the sheets? Or maybe you make Miss Manners look like an amateur. Find out if your bedroom etiquette passes the white glove test.

1. **Your guy goes limp as soon as you both get naked. You:**
   a. Act like he's hard as a rock.
   b. Announce that you're no longer interested, thanks to his wet noodle.
   c. Help him get it up again.

2. **In the heat of the moment, you shout out your old boyfriend's name. You:**
   a. Shut your mouth and hope he didn't notice.
   b. Quickly switch to the new guy's name.
   c. Keep repeating your old boyfriend's name.

3. **His caresses make you feel about as electric as a dead lightbulb. You:**
   a. Gently show his hands and mouth what to do.
   b. Pretend that he is turning you on, and moan to prove it.
   c. Tell him to stop—because he's as clumsy as a clown.

4. **His condom breaks. What to do?**
   a. Clean up and buy a pregnancy test tomorrow.
   b. Act like you didn't notice.
   c. Inform him that he better be ready to take responsibility for the kid.

5. **He's waiting in bed and you've just gone to slip into something more comfortable. Drat, your period has started. What to do?**
   a. Explain in vulgar detail why you are no longer interested.
   b. Tell him you don't mind blood on the sheets.
   c. Ignore it and hope you don't make a mess.

6. **He starts to kiss you, but his ripe breath makes you gag. You:**
   a. Scream that he has dog breath and needs to use some Listerine, now.
   b. Discreetly plug your nose and continue.
   c. Ask him what he had for dinner.

7. **Moments before penetration, you realize that you need to go to the bathroom. You:**
   a. Hold it.
   b. Excuse yourself, then slip into the bathroom.
   c. Jump out of bed and inform him you have to do number 1, and probably even number 2.

8. **Your roommate walks in on you and your date in a compromising position. You:**
   a. Shout, "Oh, not again!"
   b. Wave her out of the room.
   c. Pray she turns around.

9. **Your neighbors pound on the wall, thanks to all the noise you two are making. You:**
   a. Laugh and continue.
   b. Quiet down, and hope he hushes up too.
   c. Pound back and tell them to get a life.

10. **His nails are too long for your comfort. You:**
    a. Grin and bear it.
    b. Tell him you didn't think you were going to bed with Edward Scissorhands.
    c. Encourage him to move beyond just touching and later throw some nail clippers in his gym bag.

11. **You discover he has back hair, your pet peeve. You:**
    a. Shout "Gross!" as soon as you see it. Then banish him from your bedroom.
    b. Avoid touching his back at all costs.
    c. Send him a brochure from a salon that offers waxings.

12. **He suggests a position that frightens you. What to do?**
    a. Don't let him see your tears.
    b. Propose a different way.
    c. Tell him that only serial killers do it that way.

Scoring
```
 1. a–1   b–3   c–2
 2. a–1   b–2   c–3
 3. a–2   b–1   c–3
 4. a–2   b–1   c–3
 5. a–3   b–2   c–1
 6. a–3   b–1   c–2
 7. a–1   b–2   c–3
 8. a–3   b–2   c–1
 9. a–2   b–1   c–3
10. a–1   b–3   c–2
11. a–3   b–1   c–2
12. a–1   b–2   c–3
```

30 points or more: Howard Stern

You are as blunt as the talk show host. That's part of why your man likes you. But too brash and too bold doesn't always cut it in the bedroom. James Sniechowski, Ph.D.—half of the husband-wife psychology team who wrote *The New Intimacy: Discovering the Magic at the Heart of Your Differences* (Health Communications)—says, "Miss Blunt is profoundly caught up in some kind of fantasy. You are deeply self-involved. You tell yourself 'but I'm just telling the truth' and have no respect for the impact your words have. In the end, you will not be understood or cared for, and won't understand why." How to fix your harsh ways? Dr. Sniechowski's wife and partner, Judith Sherven, Ph.D., says, "You need to look at your unconscious need to sabotage your relationships. Is there a pattern of being overly blunt and abrasive?" Her husband adds, "The very least you can do when you feel the impulse to tell the truth in your way is to stop. Out of that will emerge a way of behaving that will be more beneficial to you."

20 to 29 points: Emily Post

Your mother taught you well—your manners are impeccable. She showed you how to behave at the table, and you've figured out how those rules apply elsewhere. Whatever blunder takes place in the bedroom, you smooth it over and get back to the good stuff. Dr. Sherven says, "You are mature, respectful, and self-respecting. But there is still room for you to become even more open, more direct." Try telling him—in a caring, respectful way—that he needs to use the Listerine you left out for him.

19 points or fewer: Scaredy-Cat

Perhaps your parents got really mad at you when you spilled your milk. Or maybe you never turned a glass over, and so now you don't know what to do when you encounter a mess. Either way, you pretend that something embarrassing or difficult isn't happening when it is. "You might justify your behavior by calling it sensitive or patient or kind," says Dr. Sniechowski. But, says Dr. Sherven, "For you to have love or even just sexual satisfaction, you are going to have to take risks." What to do? Dr. Sherven says, "You need to understand that it is not your job to make sure that everything is perfectly comfortable and nice. Then you can have a more mature relationship." So go on, let him know what you like in bed—as well as what really turns you off.✳

How Bare Do You Dare?

Are you modest and meek or dying to streak? Take *Cosmo*'s quiz to see whether you need to adjust your nude attitude.

1. **You and your friends are on a lingerie excursion. First item up for grabs: a sequined thong. Your response:**
   a. No way. You want as much cotton coverage as possible. Live by the Loom, die by the Loom.
   b. Thong shmong. Why not save money and go naked as always?
   c. Ante up. Nothing like a little undercover naughtiness to spice up your day.

2. **After working out, your locker room routine is to:**
   a. Change out of your sweaty clothes in the bathroom stall so no one gets a glimpse of your goodies.
   b. Quickly hop out of the shower and avoid conversation until you've put on your bra and panties.
   c. Stretch, apply a full face of makeup, and discuss the latest episode of *Ally McBeal* with your neighbors—au naturel.

3. **You take the day to go swimsuit shopping and are forced to change in a communal dressing room. You:**
   a. Happily strip, then ask fellow shoppers, "Do my nipples look weird to you?"
   b. Undress as if you were alone but keep your eyes on your own prizes.
   c. Try the suit on over your regular clothes. You're not about to show your skin to a bunch of bargain biddies at Loehmann's.

4. **You're about to do serious sack time with your new man. While he preps the bed, you:**
   a. Immediately unleash your assets and purr, "Feast your eyes on *these* babies!"
   b. Emerge in your favorite cotton jammies. When things get really crazy, you'll let him undo the flap.

c. Peel off your clothes to reveal your sexiest bra and panty set. He can take it from there.

5. Your sister tells you that she and her husband are going on a nudist retreat. You:
a. Reply, "That's great!" then call your mom to let her know that she raised a pervert.
b. Are happy for her—just as long as you don't have to sit though a slide show when they come back.
c. Scoff, "Who needs a retreat?" You do the backyard in the buff whenever the mood strikes you.

6. After one too many drinks at a party, the host suggests a midnight skinny-dip. You:
a. Feign a communicable disease and make tracks to the nearest exit.
b. Cheer them on, but keep your clothes and your dignity intact.
c. Streak to the pool screaming, "Last one in is a rotten egg!"

7. You're watching an indie flick with a first date when the lead actor drops his pants and gives the audience the full monty. You:
a. Immediately rush to the candy counter for more Jujyfruits—whether you're hungry for them or not.
b. Cringe a little and feel thankful that the lights are low to cover your momentary blushing.
c. Remark loudly, "I've seen bigger."

8. While visiting your parents, you unexpectedly walk in on your father—completely naked. You:
a. Commence therapy. Seeing the equipment of your origin is too much for you to endure without the help of a trained professional.
b. Immediately shut the door and apologize. Yes, going through life without seeing your father's "family tree" would have been ideal, but you can put it behind you.
c. Aren't a bit fazed. You've seen plenty of naked men before.

9. Your best friend confides in you that she once worked as a topless dancer to earn extra cash in college. You:
a. Pity her. The *real* money was in the bottomless industry.
b. Are appalled. Why didn't she just sell crack to schoolchildren?
c. Probe her for a few details but then drop the topic. The past is the past.

10. **After a dinner party with friends, someone suggests a game of strip poker. You:**

    a. Lose on purpose. When *you're* nude—everybody wins.

    b. Agree, but not before you put your coat, gloves, and hat back on.

    c. Go for it—just as long as you don't have to go past your skivvies.

Scoring

1. a–0   b–2   c–1
2. a–0   b–1   c–2
3. a–2   b–1   c–0
4. a–2   b–0   c–1
5. a–0   b–1   c–2
6. a–0   b–1   c–2
7. a–0   b–1   c–2
8. a–0   b–1   c–2
9. a–2   b–0   c–1
10. a–2   b–0   c–1

16 points or more: Brazen Bare-Ass

An orangutan has more inhibitions than you. You simply don't understand why so many people have a cover-up complex. Happy to bare your wares at the slightest provocation, your unabashed behavior puts you somewhere between *Penthouse* and *National Geographic*. In fact, your clothing-optional comfort level is on the exhibitionist end of the skin-revealing scale. "You flaunt your outside because you're afraid of revealing what's on the inside," says Katie Arons, author of *Sexy at Any Size* (Simon & Schuster). That's not to say that pride in one's appearance is a mark against you. But if bare-assed is the only way you can bear to be, then your au naturel actions reveal more about you than your butt cheeks. "As a child, you may have not been valued on the basis of your talents and abilities so you looked to your appearance to give you the recognition that you needed," says Arons. Add that to the thrill you got by shocking others with your exhibitionism and *viola!* a flesh-flaunting fetish was born. So what in fact may appear as *Uber* self-confidence may actually be a cry for acceptance from the people around you. How can you break free from your "dare to bare" mentality? "The key is to base your worth on something other than your appearance," says Arons. Set goals in life that reflect something other than what you see in the mirror every day. People will pay attention to you when you're wearing more than your bra and panties if you say or do something worthwhile. By focusing in on the things you can control in this world, you'll suffer less when those ever precious assets inevitably head south.

8 to 15 points: Semi-Buff Babe

You're no nude prude—you're not afraid to take it off when the time is right. Then again, you know that an okay body image isn't necessarily equated with swiveling around a pole in your birthday suit. You have an appreciation of the human body in all its fleshy forms, but you know where to draw the line between Amish and *Oh my gosh!* "Your parents probably accepted you as is," says Arons, and as a result, you've been able to dodge the confidence killers that can sideswipe a good self-image but haven't had to resort to buck-naked behavior to get noticed. Just maintain the balance between your self-image and the mirror-image, and you'll probably always like what you see both in and out of your clothes.

7 points or fewer: Buttoned-up Bore

No nude is good nude as far as you're concerned. You see shedding clothes as shameful rather than accepting nakedness as a normal, natural human state, and with your skewed nude view comes a plethora of problems involving body image, sexuality, and human nature in general. In fact, just the thought of having to take it off can send you into puritanical panic, fearful that someone other than your cat might see you in your God-given splendor. Not to say that you should be billboarding your boobs to strangers, but your reluctance to reveal can be almost as stifling as the turtleneck pajama set you wear to bed each night. "Some people have negative body images because their self-perception isn't in tune with reality," says Monica Brasco, Ph.D., and author of *Never Good Enough: Freeing Yourself from the Chains of Perfectionism* (The Free Press). Others associate nudity with sex and that makes them uncomfortable in their birthday best. To improve your nude attitude: stop thinking of nakedness as dirty—think of it as simply part of the package of being a person. And if a beat-up body image is making you cover up, take a good look around you. "In the real world most women don't fit those cookie-cutter images you see in the media," says Arons. "So why should you be expected to meet such strict standards?" Once you accept others in all stages of undress, you'll become as comfortable in your skin as you are in that flannel jumper.✳

Dare to Bare Do's and Don'ts

Do: Wear that sexy new dress with the plunging neckline to a romantic dinner with your man.
Don't: Wear a see-through gauze top—sans bra—to his parents' house for Thanksgiving dinner.

Do: Prance around the house wearing nothing but a smile the next time your honey comes over.
Don't: Extend the same courtesy to the pizza delivery boy.

Do: Wear an Elizabeth Hurleyesque nightie gown to the hottest club in town.
Don't: Wear it to work on casual Friday.

Do: Show off your brand-new tattoo—a butterfly on your right "cheek"—in that string bikini you bought.
Don't: Say "look what I did last night" and flash it from under your G-string to your boss.

Do: Listen to your mother and bundle up with lots of layers in the winter.
Don't: Wear your long johns under your sweats under your flannel pj's when your new man comes over for a romantic dinner.

Do: Choreograph a sexy little striptease for your stud.
Don't: Repeat it on the table of a nice restaurant after having one too many drinks.

Do: Take sexy centerfold photos to stuff in your Santa's stocking.
Don't: Post them on the Internet.

Will Your Sex Life Sizzle Forever or Fizzle Fast?

The two of you are hotter than Aruba in July. You make *9½ Weeks* look like *Toy Story*. This is definitely the best sex you've ever had. But can it last? Take this quiz and find out.

1. **On Sunday mornings the both of you:**
   a. Are still in the body pretzel you were making Saturday night.
   b. Take a hiatus from your so-so simmer to meet friends for brunch.
   c. Break out the hymnals—time to cleanse yourself of impure thoughts.

2. **In the middle of sex, you:**
   a. Count the ceiling tiles.
   b. Don't want it to end.
   c. Wonder if he noticed your flabby ass.

3. **When *he* has an orgasm he:**
   a. Pats you on the head and says, "Good job, kid."
   b. Makes sure you've peaked to perfection as well.
   c. Hopes you don't walk in and catch him.

4. **After sex there's:**
   a. Snuggling.
   b. Snoring.
   c. Skid marks.

5. **One moonlit night at the beach he spontaneously strips and runs in the water. You:**
   a. Are right beside him.
   b. Hesitate, but jump in.
   c. Are confused. It's a children's beach.

6. **When you describe him to your friends, you tell them to think of:**
   a. David Duchovny.
   b. David Schwimmer.
   c. David Koresh.

7. **After a weekend sex marathon, he:**
   a. Says, "See ya next weekend!"
   b. Is out 500 bucks. Heidi Fleiss doesn't take IOUs.
   c. Thinks he's in love.

8. **After all this sex, you know his:**
   a. Astrological sign, alma mater, and e-mail address.
   b. Middle name, favorite color, and who he took to the prom.
   c. Back has way too much hair.

9. **The both of you decide to go away together for the weekend. Your idea of the perfect getaway has:**
   a. No phone, no TV, and a king-size bed.
   b. Decent accommodations and plenty of outdoor activities.
   c. HBO.

10. **You call his house in the morning and a woman answers the phone. You:**
    a. Exclaim, "Who the hell are you?"
    b. Reply, "Uh, this is the VD clinic. Is Tom available?"
    c. Ask for him politely. It could be his sister.

Scoring

1. a–2   b–1   c–0
2. a–0   b–2   c–1
3. a–2   b–1   c–0
4. a–2   b–1   c–0
5. a–2   b–1   c–0
6. a–2   b–1   c–0
7. a–1   b–0   c–2
8. a–1   b–2   c–0
9. a–2   b–1   c–0
10. a–1   b–0   c–2

16 points or more: Bright but Brief

You two do more body-slamming than the World Wrestling Federation. There is nothing like being in a lusty, sexy relationship. Your skin glows, your body tingles, and hey—you're getting some! As long as you both are happy on a headboard-banging basis, then there's really nothing wrong with your booty-buddy lifestyle. Can it last? "In order to maintain your lusty sex life, make sure to keep things fresh. Don't be afraid to use your imagination," says Sari Locker, author of *The Complete Idiot's Guide to Amazing Sex* (Alpha). To make that flame burn even hotter, she also suggests you and your lover make a list of your top 10 sex fantasies and pick 5 that you'd like to act out.

8 to 15 points: Flickering Flame

Your bedroom relations tend to run hot and cold. Sure, sometimes the sex is okay, but there's definitely a hint that something is amiss. You may want to examine what it is that keeps interfering with your interfacing. "When the sex starts to get boring, it often means that you've fallen into a routine," says Locker. To rekindle your lustful longing, Locker's advice is to re-create a date from a time when the sex was hot and heavy, or make love in new locations, at different times of the day, and in any new positions that you can imagine. As long as you and your mate have a clear signal as to what you want out of your parallel pairing, then the two of you should get back to tearing up those sheets.

7 points or fewer: Complete and Utter Darkness

There's more sex going on at a convalescent center. Your cold-fish couplings are a sure sign that something is up. Take a long, hard look at him and yourself. What brought you two together in the first place? "When your sex life is all fizzle and no sizzle, it's a sign you are having deeper problems," says Locker. One of you may be putting some mileage on someone else's sheets, or Locker warns that a lack of sexual desire may be something to see a doctor or therapist about. But it also just might be time to face the hard, cold facts: You're meant to move on and hook hips with an equally horny honey. If he's a loser both horizontally and vertically, then maybe you should make tracks rather than make love. ✳

Are You a Tease**?**

Do you bring men to the brink only to knock 'em down domino style? Take this quiz to see if you're tempt-and-take-off ways are taking their toll.

1. **Your best friend sets you up on a blind date. You wear:**
    a. Something nice but casual. You don't want to give the impression that there'll be any horizontal dancing later tonight.
    b. A low-slung top with *two* WonderBras—to make him *wonder* if he'll get some.
    c. Something inspired by the *Dr. Quinn Medicine Woman* collection. Modesty is in, you know.

2. **Your neighbor—the David Duchovny double—makes a casual comment to you about the nice weather outside. You:**
    a. Readily agree adding, "It's one of those days when you don't want to wear panties at all!"
    b. Flirt a little. "It's so beautiful, I'll probably take a dip in the pool later."
    c. Thwart his potential advance by saying, "Yeah, but it really brings out the weirdos," as you nod in his direction.

3. **While on vacation, a sexy lifeguard begins flirting with you. Your response?**
    a. Give him a coy smile and return to your book.
    b. Ask him to rub a little lotion on your back, then tell him to get lost.
    c. Ask the name of his supervisor and have him fired.

4. **That gorgeous UPS man shows up at your door with a delivery. You:**
    a. Purr, "That's quite a *package* you've got there"—sign for it, then shut the door on him.
    b. Offer him a glass of water, wave a friendly good-bye, then vow to order half the Victoria's Secret catalogue by next week.

c. Peek from behind the curtain and demand he leave it on the doorstep. That will put the parcel pervert in his place.

5. **While driving to your boyfriend's house, the guy in the car next to you gives you a smile and a wink. You:**
    a. Roll down your windows and reply, "my headlights put the car's to shame"—then peel out of sight.
    b. Offer a smile and drive on.
    c. Look him straight in the eye, mouth "I have herpes," and watch the smoke trail form.

6. **On an outing with the girls, you get approached by an intriguing stranger. Problem? You're engaged. You:**
    a. Make conversation but subtly interject a line about your fiancé.
    b. Mention your impending vows only after you're sure you've reeled him in.
    c. Brush him off. An engaged woman shouldn't be consorting with men in public.

7. **You're having a little after-date couch play and about to reach the point of no return. You:**
    a. See if he has any condoms. You're obviously about to get down to business.
    b. Try out the knee-in-the-groin self-defense trick you've just learned to shut him down.
    c. See if he has any sandwich fixings. You're hungry all of a sudden.

8. **While sitting in a darkened theater, you reach for the popcorn and accidentally brush *his* kernels.**
    a. Apologize quickly and turn red as a beet.
    b. Do it several more times for fun—even though you know he won't get anywhere later.
    c. Accuse him of the old hand-to-the-penis popcorn trick and storm out of the theater.

9. **A platonic male friend sheepishly inquires if your ample bosom is man-made. You:**
    a. Give him a quick tweak, then let him decide for himself.
    b. Inquire incredulously, "You've thought about my breasts?"
    c. Tell him some things are better left a mystery.

10. **Your best friend is out of town and asks you to keep her boyfriend company. You:**
   a. Agree. He can help you decide which leopard-print panties to buy.
   b. Refuse. You know a bad situation when you see one.
   c. Comply. A little lunch together won't hurt.

Scoring

1. a–2 b–1 c–0
2. a–2 b–1 c–0
3. a–1 b–2 c–0
4. a–2 b–1 c–0
5. a–2 b–1 c–0
6. a–1 b–2 c–0
7. a–1 b–0 c–2
8. a–1 b–2 c–0
9. a–2 b–0 c–1
10. a–2 b–0 c–1

16 points or more: Tawdry Temptress
You do more taking back than Wal-Mart after Christmas. Using your booty as bounty, you put it out, then pull it back, leaving the men around you almost as confused as they are painfully aroused. "You doubt your desirability," says Sari Locker, author of *The Complete Idiot's Guide to Amazing Sex* (Alpha), "so you have to prove it over and over again by leading guys on and watching them fall." But that carrot-dangling attitude is putting more out on the line than just your unattainable jewels. "By never following through, you'll start to lose respect from the people around you and likely get kicked curbside after one too many games," says Locker. So what do you do if you can't resist bringing him to the edge, then opting out? "You need to take an honest look at your actions," says Locker. When you find yourself brushing his arm or laughing at his lame jokes, recognize and walk away. Simple as that. Also, learn to invest in some alone time. Get a hobby or indulge in a favorite activity— solo. Once you learn that being alone isn't the most horrible thing in the world, you'll be less likely to engage in your trick-or-treat behavior.

8 to 15 points: Give-and-Take Gal

You're a woman of your word. You know where you stand and, more important, where and when you lay—and so do the people around you. "Your parents likely instilled in you the confidence to make your own decisions," says Mira Kirshenbaum, author of *Women & Love* (Avon). So you trust that inner voice that rarely waivers when it comes to big decisions—and that includes with whom and when you slap skins. You get no kicks out of taking people for a ride; rather, you lay the cards on the table because you're comfortable with the hand you've been dealt. "You know the value of intimacy and understand that feelings are not to be toyed with," says Locker. In fact, you're so self-assured, you prefer to focus on your personal achievements—none of which include the trail of broken hearts you've left behind. So just keep your bounds of mutual respect clear as they have been in the past and you're sure to have similar success in the future. And remember, what goes around comes around. By radiating the vibes of respect and love, you're guaranteed to always get it back tenfold.

7 points or fewer: Cross-legged Coward

You're about one step away from wearing a belt emblazoned with "Do Not Enter." Unlike the tease who employs a maybe-you-will, maybe-you-won't mentality, you've padlocked your panties and pulled a sexual shutdown. Not only do you not tease, you're happy to lash out Xena-style at anyone who dares to regard you as a sexual being. "You may have had a very negative situation with a man, whether it be abuse or rejection, when you were young, which makes you want to avoid them all together," says Kirshenbaum. Or perhaps your parents or your religious influences lead you to believe that women should not express their desire to have sex. In any case, the result is a sexually stunted attitude that can halt intimacy right in its tracks. "It's okay to respect your boundaries, but realize that sex isn't a dirty word," says Kirshenbaum. Try to debunk those negative sexual myths by discussing your carnal conundrum with friends whose opinions you respect. Once you get a handle on your sexually skewed view, you can set that inner vixen free.✳

What Kind of Sexual Vibe
Do You Give Off ?

Is your calendar blooming with dates, dotted with one-night stands, or withering from man-drought? Maybe it's your vibe. Find out what kind you're sending out.

1. You're deep in conversation at a party when the hostess interrupts to introduce you to a *majorly* handsome man. Naturally, you:
- a. Maneuver him away from every other single woman in the room.
- b. Smile, touch his arm, and ask his opinion on the topic at hand.
- c. Return to your conversation as soon as the introductions are over.

2. When your lover mentions your clothes, it's usually to say:
- a. "Why don't you wear something to show off your nice body for a change?"
- b. "Do you expect me to spend the night fighting off every guy in town?"
- c. "Babe, you look great as usual!"

3. It's your first dinner out with a man, and so far the evening's been terrific. When the waiter brings the dessert menu to the table, you:
- a. Order decaf. You have to work early tomorrow, and you never indulge in sweets.
- b. Suggest your date come back for "something really sweet" at your place.
- c. Choose a gooey dessert that you can share—1 dish and 2 forks!

4. You wear your nails:
- a. Painted the hottest color of the week.
- b. Long and talonlike, so a man can imagine them scratching his back.
- c. Clipped and colorless.

5. When it comes to drinking at big parties, you always:
- a. Stay far away from the bar; you like to be in absolute and total control.
- b. Have a couple of shots of tequila with lime—how else can you get the nerve to jump up on the bar and do the Macarena?

> Standing tall, looking him straight in the eye, showing a sense of humor—these are key in letting a man know you're available but not giving it away.

c. Nurse 1 or 2 drinks—*if* you need a little loosening up.

6. **Which of these quotes could have come out of *your* mouth?**
   a. "Life is a banquet—and most poor suckers are starving."
      —*Rosalind Russell as Auntie Mame*
   b. "I've been in more laps than a napkin."
      —*Mae West*
   c. "Sex is a bad thing, because it rumples the clothes."   —*Jackie O.*

7. **You keep a stash of condoms in:**
   a. A crystal dish on a living room table.
   b. In your purse, and cleverly secreted around your apartment.
   c. The medicine cabinet—behind the toothpaste, Band-Aids, alcohol, and cotton balls.

8. **When it comes to disclosing your deepest intimacies, you:**
   a. Love to talk. No subject should be taboo.
   b. Reveal almost nothing—unless you're confessing to your priest.
   c. Save the really juicy material for your shrink and *closest* friends.

9. **To the gym, you wear:**
   a. Dark sweatpants and a T-shirt.
   b. Bike shorts and a muscle T-shirt.
   c. A tight thong leotard over flesh-tone tights—and makeup, of course.

10. **Check any of the statements that most apply to you:**
    a. You're comfortable telling a lover what feels good—and what doesn't.
    b. You close the door to the bathroom—even when no one else is home.
    c. You'd need at least 2 hands to count the one-night stands you've had.
    d. You'd never use sex to win a client—though you're not above employing a snug above-the-knee suit.
    e. All your necklaces strategically hit the top of your always visible cleavage.
    f. You never look strangers in the eye.
    g. You don't stop flirting with a man even after he's fallen in love with you.

Scoring

1. a–3   b–2   c–1
2. a–1   b–3   c–2
3. a–1   b–3   c–2
4. a–2   b–3   c–1
5. a–1   b–3   c–2
6. a–2   b–3   c–1
7. a–3   b–2   c–1
8. a–3   b–1   c–2
9. a–1   b–2   c–3
10. Give yourself 1 point each for *b, f*. Give yourself 2 points each for *a, d, g*. Give yourself 3 points each for *c, e*.

Fewer than 24 points: Chilly Chick

As much as you want to share an intimate moment with that handsome new man, whenever he looks your way, you avert your eyes or simply turn your back. Uncomfortable in clothes that show off your figure, you hide yourself in dark colors and businesslike suits.

So, how can you defrost? Start by reaching out: "The cold woman has a tendency to close people out," says Susan Block, Ph.D., author of *The Ten Commandments of Pleasure* (St. Martin's Press). "A way to counteract that is to become a more active listener. Pretend that you're going to be tested on what you hear." And don't *you* forget to open up: "Try taking small steps at first," says Block. "Start low-risk conversations with people like the deli man. After a while, you can chat up someone you really care about." And don't forget to use the power of physical interaction, adds Bernie Zilbergeld, Ph.D., a sex therapist in Oakland, California: "Tapping a man on his shoulder or wrist is innocent—but also inviting and warm."

As for dress, says Block, go for the touchable: suede, silk, or leather—they are sensual against your skin and look inviting. Block suggests wearing thong underwear and push-up bras when you are going out. "A thong can be stimulating! And seeing your own cleavage reminds you you're a woman who doesn't mind being an occasional sex object."

24 to 38 points: Wanted Woman

"You are so perfectly attractive, men probably act like fools when they're with you," declares Barbara Keesling, author of *Super Sexual Orgasm* (HarperCollins). "You stand tall, make eye contact, and have a sense of humor." As for your dress sense, you know how to match the outfit to the moment—key in sending out a message that says you're available but not for hire, says Block.

This understanding of what's appropriate extends to your dating life. Confident he will call again, you would never lure a new man with sexual favors, say Marcia and Lisa Douglass, Ph.D.s, and authors of *Are We Having Fun Yet? The Intelligent Woman's Guide to Sex* (Hyperion). "Also, you always carry condoms, refusing to buy into the idea that nice girls don't plan for sex," say Marcia and Lisa Douglass. "Men who aren't used to women in control of their own sexuality may be threatened. But the Wanted Woman always goes for a man who will worship at her temple."

More than 38 points: Desperate Dater

You've developed a pattern of using sex as a lure, baiting your hook with cleavage and suggestive comments, tempting him with intimate touches way too early, and trying to reel him in by offering up good sex when a good-night kiss would do. You've become convinced you have nothing to offer a man other than your body. "These women think driving a man wild gives them control over him," says Block. Ah, but only for 1 or 2 nights. As Zilbergeld points out, men "rightfully figure you're like this with every guy you meet." And while they might very well take advantage of your hot loving, they're usually gone by daybreak, leaving you even more desperate to lure a new lover boy.

To stop the endless cycle of one-night stands, first *calm down* says Zilbergeld. "Take up some form of meditation. It can help you become more comfortable with yourself and this will help alleviate your constant anxiety to meet someone." Next, he says, set some ground rules for yourself. If you don't yet have a sense of what is appropriate, find a friend to model yourself after.

You may also want to tap your friend for a little pre-date counseling. "Let her tell you if your dress is way too provocative," says

Sexy versus Slutty Do's and Don'ts

Do: Wear those new leather pants to your next hot dinner date.
Don't: Wear them with a halter top and stilettos.

Do: Lean into your man and whisper, "I can't wait to get you home tonight" in the middle of a dinner party.
Don't: Ask the guy you just met at the dinner party to stop by later because your boyfriend will be long gone and dessert's on you.

Do: During sex, tell him that he does things to your body that you never thought possible.
Don't: Say that the only other guy who could make you come like this is his best friend.

Do: Wear thigh-high stockings and a miniskirt—sans panties—to dinner-for-two at his place.
Don't: Wear the same thing to work, and explicitly uncross your legs to bare all during a meeting.

Do: Wear the perfect shade of traffic—stopping red lipstick with your elegant black suit.
Don't: Tease your hair, add lots of black eye makeup, and lose the suit in favor of Daisy Dukes.

Block, who also advises giving yourself a 1-drink maximum for the night. "Some of these women are getting drunk at parties or on dates and acting in ways they might not if they were sober." Finally, try cloaking yourself in a little mystery: "Don't let these guys know every sexual encounter you have had," says Block. "The guy you're meeting at a bar is not your best friend—not yet, anyway." ✳

Do: Make the most of your Marilyn Monroe–curves with sexy and simple 50s-style halter dresses.
Don't: Buy the dress 2 sizes too small and wear a WonderBra so that your breasts are at chin level.

Do: Make sure your nails are perfectly polished with whatever color suits your mood this week.
Don't: Wear your nails so long that they look like they belong on an endangered species.

How Adventurous Are You in Bed?

If you want a scintillating sex life, you've got to be a rule-breaker in bed. And in the bathtub. And on the kitchen table. But can increasingly over-the-top lovemaking be big-time bad news? Take this quiz to find out if you're going too far when getting it on.

1. **Your lover playfully spanks you during foreplay. Your reaction?**
   a. You laugh and squeal, "Punish me! I've been a very bad girl."
   b. Not applicable. You always lie flat on your back, so he never touches your tush.
   c. You grab your riding crop, pin him down, and say, "If you're going to spank me, honey, you better do it right."

2. **The ideal threesome in bed is:**
   a. You, your man, and a well-chosen trinket from a sex catalog.
   b. You, Antonio Sabáto, Jr., and Xena, warrior princess.
   c. You, a book, and a cup of herbal tea.

3. **You make love in the dark:**
   a. Always, so your partner can't see your flab wobbling all over the place.
   b. Sometimes, since feeling your way around in bed can be erotic.
   c. Never, unless you count being blindfolded or doing it outside at night.

4. **Your lover is into the uptight-librarian-who-takes-off-her-glasses-and-lets-down-her-hair-to-unleash-the-slut-within fantasy. You:**
   a. Put your hair in a bun and ask what he'd like to "check out" (wink, wink).
   b. Grab your library card, head to your local branch, and do it with him Dewey decimal–style in the stacks.
   c. Refer him to the self-help section—because he needs it, bad.

5. **Have you ever sucked on someone's toes?**
   a. Sure—and that's just one of many tootsie turn-ons. . . .
   b. Yes, but only after he's showered and scrubbed away any sock funk.
   c. Ugh! Never. Can you say *foot fungus*?

6. **Midsex, you might say:**
   a. "Mmmm, baby, that feels *so* good."
   b. "Ouch! You're squashing my arm."
   c. "Faster! Harder! More! MORE!"

7. **A girlfriend asks you to accompany her to an upscale sex shop. You leave with:**
   a. A bottle of massage oil and a couple of wilder goodies.
   b. A shopping bag full of orgasmic trinkets and some bondage gear.
   c. A sick feeling in your stomach over the moral decay of society.

8. **Do you masturbate?**
   a. Yes
   b. No

9. **One-night stands are:**
   a. A perfectly legitimate way to salvage a sucky Saturday night.
   b. Not your norm, but you've been known to get swept away on occasion.
   c. Nasty, sexually transmitted disasters that are just waiting to happen.

10. **Congratulations! You're having an orgasm. Who knows about it?**
   a. No one—you're much too embarrassed to make a sound.
   b. Your partner—you love letting him know when he's rocked your world.
   c. The neighbors and anyone who happens to be within a 3-block radius of your house.

11. **Your man wants to watch a porn flick with you. What do you think?**
   a. Why bother? It will be more fun to grab the camcorder and make our own!
   b. Why not? It could be a trashy turn-on, as long as it's not violent or offensive.
   c. Why me? I always wind up with these sicko perverts.

12. **Have you ever had sex (circle all that apply):**
   a. In a car?
   b. In a movie theater?
   c. At your parents' house—while they were home?

d. Near a window with the blinds up?
e. In the bathtub/shower?
f. In a closet, coatroom, etc., at a party?
g. While a third person was in the room?
h. In front of a video camera?

Scoring

1. a–2   b–1   c–3
2. a–2   b–3   c–1
3. a–1   b–2   c–3
4. a–2   b–3   c–1
5. a–3   b–2   c–1
6. a–2   b–1   c–3
7. a–2   b–3   c–1
8. Yes, 3; No, 1
9. a–3   b–2   c–1
10. a–1   b–2   c–3
11. a–3   b–2   c–1
12. 1–2 circled answers: 1 point; 3–5 answers: 2 points; 6 or more: 3 points

29 points or more: Voracious Vixen

You're a gymnastic, multiorgasmic dynamo, so take pride in your adventurous attitude. "You know what gives you pleasure and aren't afraid to ask for it," says Stella Resnick, Ph.D., a psychologist in Los Angeles and author of *The Pleasure Zone: Why We Resist Good Feelings and How to Let Go and Be Happy* (Conari Press). "Many women are too shy to do that," she says.

Just make sure that your quest for kink is not a substitute for emotional intimacy. "Sex in a close relationship is psychologically, spiritually, and physically the most amazing thing on earth," says Joel Block, Ph.D., a clinical psychologist in Huntington, New York, and author of *The Romance of Sex* (Parker Publishing). That may explain why—if you engage in multiple sex-a-thons with people you don't care about—you may find yourself emotionally unsatisfied, says Resnick. Try exploring your sensual side with one special man. "Taste the wine on his lips, feel the goose bumps that rise when skin slides on skin," Block suggests, as these subtle sensual acts are ways of being intimate—not just getting off. If getting close

holds no appeal, or if you can't stop yourself from pursuing promiscuous, anonymous, and/or unsafe sex, talk to a therapist, because risking every-thing for an orgasmic rush could be a sign of sexual addiction. Otherwise, celebrate your buckwild libido—safely, of course.

21 to 28 points: Naughty and Nice
The perfect balance of raunch and restraint, you are open to creative coupling, but you know that not every encounter has to be a superfreaky chandelier-swinger. "The more you and your partner know about each other, the more you'll please each other," explains Block. "If you're lucky, your desires will coincide with your partner's. But even if they don't always, they may stimulate new ideas that you both want to try."

Most important, your spirit of experimentation will head off bed-room ruts. "You won't lose interest in your partner, because sex for you never stops being inventive," says Resnick. But if the fireworks fade, don't panic. As long as you let your lover know your wants, needs, and secret fantasies, you'll get back into the sexual swing of things.

20 points or fewer: Repressed Princess
You are a desirable, passionate woman who can—and deserves to—feel the earth move. Unfortunately, you have a play-by-the-rules

"The Wildest Thing I've Ever Done"

"My boyfriend and I drove cross-country and had sex in the capital cities of all the states we passed through! It made the trip a hell of a lot more fun!"
—Tara, 29, musician

"One night in college, I got really trashed—and horny—at a friend's party. I saw this guy I was secretly hot for, walked up to him, and said, 'I want to show you something.' I led him to the bathroom, locked the door, and attacked him. We did it standing up, slamming against the door while about half a dozen people waited on line right outside!"
—Cydney, 24, grad student

"I was dating a cowboy who was competing in several rodeos over the July 4th weekend last year, and I went with him. On the 4th itself, all the motels in town were booked. We wound up frolicking on the flat roof of a one-story building on Main Street as the Independence Day celebrants crammed the street right below us. It was insane."—Mari, 40, nurse

"I was feeling neglected, so I got my hair and makeup done really sexy. Then I put on a bustier and garters and spiked heels and a raincoat over them. I walked into my boyfriend's office, and let my raincoat fall open. As he tried to finish his phone call, I ran my hands all over my body. We wound up having sex in the car."
—Casey, 26, homemaker

approach to sex, which means you're missing out on scintillating experiences. You probably don't lack physical desire. "If you stop yourself from being pleasured in bed, chances are that your first sexual experiences weren't positive ones," says Resnick. It might not have been as traumatic as childhood sexual abuse—you could've simply lost your virginity to an insensitive, inept jerk. Or perhaps your parents' "don't ask, don't tell" attitude about sex has made it difficult for you to express your needs without feeling shame. "Many sex-shy women are simply afraid of what will happen if they lose all control," says Resnick.

Whatever the reason, if you'd like to have a fuller love life, you need to welcome sex as a positive thing. Start reaching out and grabbing your own pleasure. Reenacting 9½ Weeks isn't for everybody, but playful, risqué romancing can take your relationships to a whole new level. Take a candlelit bubble bath, play strip poker, savor every moment with him. If you find you can't, perhaps you don't feel safe sharing your body and mind with your partner. "Remember that sex is a healthy manifestation of the intense feelings you have for your lover," says Block. "Find someone with whom you feel comfortable enough to go wild. Life's too short for lack-luster lovemaking.✳

Cosmo's
Sexual Aptitude Test

Can the wrong medicine make you feel frigid? Could his lip sores become your vaginal nightmare? Take our test and learn what you need to know before you head for bed.

1. Your lover, a skilled oral technician, is prone to cold sores. Should it stop him from going down on you?
   a. Yes. Performing oral sex on you can make his cold sore sting.
   b. Yes. The same virus that causes sores on *his* mouth can take up residence in *your* genitals.
   c. No. Cold sores are noncontagious.

Sex-Smart Answer: b
An oral cold sore is actually an infection from the herpes virus. Granted, herpes simplex type 1 prefers to wreak havoc on the mouth, and type 2 likes to make trouble between your legs, but "if your partner has a cold sore and performs oral sex, he can transmit the type-1 virus to your genital region," says Marshall Glover, director of the Centers for Disease Control National STD hot line. So don't mix cold sores and cunnilingus.

2. *Whoopee!* You received a postcard in today's mail reminding you of your annual gyno exam. When's the best time to make the appointment?
   a. Right before your period, so she can see you in full-on PMS mode.
   b. One week after your monthly period, when all the *action* has ended.
   c. When your doc can squeeze you in.

Sex-Smart Answer: b
Schedule your appointment for about 7 days after the crimson tide has gone out. "Pap tests are easier to read when there is no blood blocking the view of the cells," says Paula E. Szypko, M.D., a

spokesperson for College of American Pathologists. Your breasts are also at their least tender and lumpy between periods. Make a point to avoid having sex or using a spermicide, vaginal lubricant, or douche 48 hours before your exam. "All those things muddy the waters, so to speak," says Dr. Szypko. And if you think you may be at risk for an STD, tell your doctor: a Pap smear only checks for abnormalities that may lead to cervical cancer—not STDs.

3. Your lover wants you to take the latter option in your ongoing spit-or-swallow debate. What's the lowdown on going down?
   a. Semen is very high in calories and fat—like a shot of Crisco.
   b. It's chock-full of vitamins and minerals that add luster to your hair and skin.
   c. It's actually effective protection against a pregnancy-related disease.

Sex-Smart Answer: c
Semen is low in fat, and an average teaspoon-size serving has less than 25 calories. Its main ingredients are water, sugars, and—oh yeah—about 100 million sperm. It's those tiny DNA missiles that might actually protect you against a common pregnancy-related disease called preeclampsia. Doctors believe this potentially dangerous disease is a reaction to your mate's proteins in the placenta, which can result in high blood pressure and premature delivery. "Prolonged exposure to the father's sperm can reduce a woman's risk," says Gustaaf Dekker, M.D., a Dutch researcher who recently completed a study of the interaction.

The rumor that semen is good for the hair and skin? A myth. It does contain traces of vitamin C and zinc—but if you relied on semen to fulfill your RDAs, you'd never be able to come up for air.

4. Your lover has broken through 3 condoms this week. Could rubbers be too small to handle the magnitude of his manhood?
   a. Yes. Even average-size guys can be too anaconda for certain brands.
   b. No. He must be using them wrong.
   c. Yes. He puts Dirk Diggler to shame—there's *no* rubber that can hold him.

Sex-Smart Answer: a or b
If a brand-new, properly cared-for condom breaks at the most inopportune moment, it *could* be because it's too small. "Not all con-

doms are created equal," says James Trussell, Ph.D., director of the Office of Population Research at Princeton University. Some luxury condoms from foreign countries are scaled down. So if it's an overseas brand he's wearing that breaks, he should try switching to a rubber made in the United States.

If your lover busts through American-made condoms, though, check the wrapper. If the date on the wrapper harkens back more than 2 years, the condom may have begun to deteriorate. And make sure to use a water-based lubricant like Astroglide: dry condoms break more easily, and oil-based lubes like Vaseline can weaken any love sleeve.

5. **Sometimes, when your lover rubs your clitoris, you cry out in pain, not pleasure. What to do?**
 a. Give your guy a sex lesson.
 b. Use some K-Y jelly.
 c. Get a little genital R&R.

Sex-Smart Answer: a, b, and c
Although men generally enjoy much rougher stimulation, the highly sensitive clitoris needs to be handled with TLC. "He's touching you the way *he* likes to be touched," says Yvonne S. Thornton, M.D., author of *Woman to Woman: A Leading Gynecologist Tells You All You Need to Know About Your Body and Your Health* (Dutton). Encourage him to pay attention to other erogenous zones—lips, breasts, earlobes, whatever makes you moist. If he starts rubbing before you're turned on, you'll feel raw—not aroused. And tell him to go a bit easier during your subsequent go-arounds. The supersensitive clitoris can only take so much without a break.

6. **For a few days between periods, you notice a brownish discharge on your panties. Should you douche and snuff the stuff at its source?**
 a. No. The vagina is like a self-cleaning oven—it doesn't need douche.
 b. Yes! Douche away that not-so-fresh feeling! You don't want nasty stuff sticking to your best lace skivvies.
 c. No. See your gyno for a Pap.

Sex-Smart Answer: a

That discharge is probably just a normal response to ovulation. About 2 weeks before your period, the ovary releases an egg, which triggers the release of more estrogen and progesterone. The vagina ups its discharge while the uterus sheds some lining and blood, all in preparation for fertilization. "These substances mix together to form what you see in your underwear," explains Dr. Thornton.

But as gross as the discharge is—as long as it doesn't smell bad and/or itch, which could indicate a vaginal infection—it's best left alone. Douching is not only unnecessary, it can leave you more susceptible to yeast infections by interfering with the good bacteria that help keep the vagina clean and healthy.

7. **You're considering various birth-control methods: the Pill, Depo-Provera shots, and Norplant. Which one might make it difficult for you to get pregnant once you stop?**
    a. Depo-Provera
    b. The Pill
    c. Norplant

Sex-Smart Answer: a

While the majority of women regain their fertility within a month of removing Norplant or going off the Pill, Depo-Provera's aftereffects can last a year—or longer. "Depo-Provera is notorious for delayed recurrence of menses," says Dr. Thornton. But later doesn't mean never: a large study of women who stopped receiving Depo-Provera injections to become pregnant found that about half of those who became pregnant did so within 10 months of their last injection; about 67 percent became pregnant within 12 months; and by the 18-month mark, 93 percent had become pregnant.

8. **You've heard that the window for getting pregnant is pretty narrow, so you sometimes skip birth control. What are your chances of getting knocked up if you do it au naturel for an entire year?**
    a. 14 percent
    b. 50 percent
    c. 85 percent

Sex-Smart Answer: c

"If you don't use birth control and aren't sterile, you're almost certain to become pregnant before the year is over," says Trussell. Using the rhythm method—not having sex leading up to and including the day of ovulation—is better but far from foolproof. You still have a 25 percent chance of becoming pregnant if that's the only method you use. "It's tough enough to judge which are those risky days, but it's even harder to have the willpower to abstain during them," says Trussell. So if you want to avoid morning sickness and all that goes with it, use your head—and protection.

9. **You think you're really turned on, but your panties are as dry as a desert. What's the problem?**
   a. It's him—there's just no sexual chemistry between you.
   b. It's you—you're obviously frigid.
   c. It's your medicine cabinet.

Sex-Smart Answer: c

Some commonly used drugs can cause a drought down below. Antihistamines, for example, found in cold remedies and allergy medications, dry out *all* your orifices—not just your nose. "Decongestants, on the other hand, can actually enhance a woman's climax," says James Goldberg, Ph.D., coauthor of *Sexual Pharmacology* (Norton). Fight back by using a generous amount of a water-based lube like Astroglide, Eros, or I-D, and by asking him to be patient! And if you're on the Pill, check the label. The progestin in some pills can cause a dry spell. Ask your doctor about switching to a pill with different levels of estrogen and progestin.✳

LIFE

Are You
High Maintenance?

Does it take the constant attention of your friends, man, and manicurist to keep you happy? Or do you have the demanding instincts of a doormat?

1. **Your guy is seriously in the mood, but you're feeling as hot as an ice-cream truck. What to do?**
   a. Ask for a back rub; that usually sparks your fire.
   b. Let him get on and get it over with.
   c. Come down with a migraine.

2. **After a hell-raising round of "Can you commit?" your man slams out the door. You:**
   a. Go solo to a movie, have coffee with a friend—anything to keep busy while you figure out what *you* want.
   b. Follow him out the door, admit you were wrong, and promise him more space than Sputnik.
   c. Bulldoze your way into all of *his* hangouts until you find him—then demand an apology.

3. **Your boss has been holed up in her office and has barely spoken to you in 3 weeks. You:**
   a. Figure she's as busy as you are.
   b. March into her office in tears, crying "I need feedback."
   c. Start looking for another job.

4. **When on a plane, how often do you buzz the flight attendant?**
   a. Never. So what if you're dying of thirst—she'll be by with the drink cart soon.
   b. Only if it's necessary, like when the drunk guy next to you passes out on your shoulder.
   c. At least 3 or 4 times—for extra pillows or blankets, lip balm, more dinner rolls . . .

5. **Your so-called friend has invited you and your two-timing ex to her party. You:**

a. Demand she disinvite him.

b. Go. Why let a jerky ex stop you from scoping better mate material?

c. Show up for hors d'oeuvres duty—staying in the kitchen to keep tensions with your former flame from boiling over into the party.

6. **Mom's latest guilt trip? "Why aren't you spending Easter with the family?" Naturally, you call your best friend and:**

a. Insist she put her romantic dinner à deux on hold so you can pump her for advice. Then you call your second-best friend and get *her* take.

b. Ask whether she's got time to give you some badly needed shrinkage.

c. Imagine the great counseling session you could have—if you could only bring yourself to burden her with tales of Mommie Dearest.

7. **The office computer system is getting upgraded Monday morning. You're so low-tech, you're still using a typewriter. How to adjust?**

a. Grab the manual and spend the weekend cramming.

b. Let some compu-nerd deal with plugging your work into the system.

c. Assume they'll have an on-site techie to help you learn the drill.

8. **A royal red zit has reared its ugly head—on the tip of your nose. You:**

a. Demand a dermatologist's appointment for that afternoon.

b. Steam and squeeze till it pops.

c. Chalk up the eruption to a premenstrual hormonal rush and forget about it.

9. **A friend calls to cancel your standing chat-and-chew night because that Brad Pitt look-alike just asked her out. Your response:**

a. Tell her she's picking up the tab for your next gab-fest.

b. Stand her up on the next go-round.

c. "Come over—I'll do your makeup."

10. **Your normally not-so-spontaneous guy tells you to put on your sexiest dress, pack a toothbrush, and meet him in an hour. You:**

a. Throw on that little black number, toss some condoms in your bag, and arrive 15 minutes early.

b. Tell him if he wants to surprise you, try 3 days' notice.

c. Take the time to choose between your Nicole Miller and Betsey Johnson, and show up 10 minutes late. You're worth the wait.

11. **Your boss throws you a major last-minute assignment. You:**
   a. Negotiate a later deadline.
   b. Demand an extra assistant—and 2 recovery days at home.
   c. Put in a 60-hour week.

12. **Your monthly beauty-health regimen includes (mark all that apply):**
   a. Manicure.
   b. Bikini wax.
   c. Bleaching/electrolysis.
   d. Massage.
   e. Yoga/meditation hour.
   f. Facial.
   g. Session with an astrologer/tarot card reader/psychic phone friend.

Scoring

 1. a–2   b–1   c–3
 2. a–2   b–1   c–3
 3. a–2   b–3   c–1
 4. a–1   b–2   c–3
 5. a–3   b–2   c–1
 6. a–3   b–2   c–1
 7. a–1   b–3   c–2
 8. a–3   b–2   c–1
 9. a–2   b–3   c–1
10. a–1   b–3   c–2
11. a–2   b–3   c–1
12. Give yourself one point for each answer checked.

30 points or more: Mistress Upkeep
Admit it: If you aren't squawking to the boss about working too hard, you're begging your boyfriend to make a midnight frozen-yogurt run. As for friends, they've learned to screen your calls, mostly to avoid hearing marathon kvetch-fests. And your pampering routine has masseuses scrambling for tickets back to Sweden.

In case you haven't figured this out, the more you ask for, the less you get, says New York City–based psychotherapist Linda Barbanel. Still, you can learn to scale back. "Wear a rubber band around your wrist, and every time you're ready to put someone out, 'snap' yourself to attention," suggests Barbanel. "Ask yourself: Do you need this favor or are you out for control, status, attention?" A self-restraining order isn't all that's required; you must also learn to give. "However much you think you give—and chances are, you think you give more than you do," says Barbanel, "double or *triple* your efforts."

20 to 29 points: Give-and-Take Girl

Do you ask a waiter to take back a funky-smelling fish dish? Of course! But with the same laid-back ease you would when asking him to recommend a Bordeaux. "This woman knows when to hold out for what she wants," says JoAnn Magdoff, a New York City–based psychotherapist, "and, as important, when to back off." You've also got finely honed payback instincts. Yes, you'll pick up your guy's dry-cleaning if he's overwhelmed at work. But you expect to be rewarded—whether it's with a half-hour back rub or dinner at your favorite sushi joint. In other words, no doormat duty for you.

19 points or fewer: Sister Self-(Dis)service

Who's asking? Certainly not you. In fact, most of your waking hours are spent satisfying everyone else's needs. And don't think this self-sacrifice is getting you voted most popular. "These women are martyrs, which is no fun at all," says Barbanel, especially in the guy department. "Being so nurturing is a turn-off; it reminds men of their mothers." Adding to your unsex-appeal: that "Why bother?" attitude when it comes to your grooming routine.

You need some "gimme" gumption. First off, "Force yourself to start making demands," says Barbanel, "even if they're small ones. Tell a friend it's her turn to cat-sit; ask your boss for more time to finish that project. You've got to trust that if you ask someone a favor, they'll oblige."

And try some self-indulgence. "Get fresh flowers," says Barbanel. "Treat yourself to expensive bath oil." Go ahead—spoil yourself a little. ✳

Do You Need an
Attitude Adjustment?

Is your attitude a turn-off? Take this quiz to find out whether your people skills need some 911 assistance.

1. Your boyfriend's mother has been planning a splashy affair for months and expects both of you to be there. The big night finds you feeling drained and cranky. You:
   a. Go with him and act charming, but let him know you need to ease out early.
   b. Go with him, grit your teeth, smile, and stay at the party until the bitter end.
   c. Decide that everyone will just have to do without you. You're putting your feet up and popping in some videos.

2. During a meeting, your assistant makes a racy wisecrack, causing higher-ups to raise their collective starchy eyebrows. You:
   a. Irritably shake your head at her and hiss, "What's wrong with you?"
   b. Pipe up, "My fault. I'm afraid I taught her everything she knows."
   c. Ignore the remark, making a mental note to later impart a few pointers about the business world to your assistant.

3. Your new man compliments you on how particularly gorgeous you look. You smile and:
   a. Reply, "Thank you."
   b. Quip, "Too bad the celebrity I resemble most is Howard Stern."
   c. Say, "I know."

4. Your superior asks you to redo a proposal drafted by a colleague. You:
   a. Accept, promising to do your best. You're happy to get a shot.
   b. Accept, adding, "But I probably won't do as good a job as she did."
   c. Roll your eyes and inform your supervisor that this is not part of your job.

> Ask a trusted friend to tell you when you're being a killjoy.

101

5. **A sudden jostle at a cocktail party sends your drink flying onto another woman's designer sheath. Anxious to right the faux pas, you:**
   a. Grab some napkins, dab the stain, and offer to pay the dry-cleaning bill.
   b. Apologize for your clumsiness.
   c. Find the person who bumped you and make sure he knows the consequences of his carelessness.

6. **In bed, your boyfriend wants you to star in an X-rated video. Not feeling particularly photogenic, you:**
   a. Acquiesce. You don't want him looking elsewhere for his leading lady.
   b. Sweetly tell him you aren't comfortable with that kind of exposure now.
   c. Let him know how disgusting you think his little fantasy is.

7. **Your supervisor criticizes a project you put your heart and soul into. Your first instinct is to:**
   a. Blame a coworker.
   b. Panic. Before you know it, you'll be out of a job and out on the street.
   c. Acknowledge the criticism—though you won't dwell on it.

8. **You forgot to call your neighbor to tell her she's left her headlights on. The next morning, a tow truck's giving her a jump start. You:**
   a. Offer her a ride to work.
   b. Apologize for your part in this fiasco, adding, "I'm such a space cadet!"
   c. Do nothing—it's her responsibility to turn her lights off. She's such a flake!

9. **Despite months of hard training for a prestigious 10K, you come in 25th. At your first chance, you'll:**
   a. Stalk icily past the winner and complain to anyone who will listen about the unfairness of it all.
   b. Simply accept the fact that you're one of life's biggest all-time losers.
   c. Congratulate the winner, and then make dinner plans with someone who you know will make you laugh.

10. **For the sixth time this week, your gal pal calls to wail to you about her loser lover. You:**
   a. Snap, "I don't have the time for this."
   b. Tell her that life can be great while you're holding out for the right man.
   c. Warn her to take the good with the bad. Available men are hard to find.

Scoring

1.	a–2	b–1	c–3
2.	a–3	b–1	c–2
3.	a–2	b–1	c–3
4.	a–2	b–1	c–3
5.	a–1	b–2	c–3
6.	a–1	b–2	c–3
7.	a–3	b–1	c–2
8.	a–2	b–1	c–3
9.	a–3	b–1	c–2
10.	a–3	b–2	c–1

Above 22: Bad Attitude

While you may think you're perfectly justified, the truth is, you're making enemies. "My first rule in life is, 'Thou shalt not burn bridges unless thou can walk on water,' " says Tina Flaherty, author of *The Savvy Woman's Success Bible* (Berkley Publishing Group). You've turned colleagues against you—mainly by being a shirker and playing the blame game. And, "for all you know, the person you offend could be very tight with the CEO," points out Flaherty. As for romance, even if "you manage to hook up with a man, he won't stay long," she says. "You're too inflexible, too 'me first.' "

This nasty attitude actually stems from a wobbly self-esteem, says Duke Robinson, author of *Good Intentions: The Nine Unconscious Mistakes of Nice People* (Warner Books). Most likely, your parents were stingy—materially, emotionally, or support-wise. So you learned to fend only for yourself—never caring whose toes you stepped on.

Upgrade your attitude by honing your people skills, "even if that means asking a trusted friend to tell you when you're being a killjoy," suggests Flaherty. You can also start focusing on making others feel good, adds Karen Salmansohn, author of *How to Succeed in Business Without a Penis* (Harmony Books). "Start seeing life from other people's points of view. And compliment, but be sincere. That will always win others over."

12 to 21 points: Good Attitude

When life throws you a curve ball, you just try to turn it into a home run. "People with good attitudes are as flexible as acrobats," says Flaherty. "If you're given an assignment at work that's not part of your job description, you accept it with gusto." Secure enough to know that being generous and kind won't cost you, you also remember to compliment friends (or even competitors) on their successes—even if your own life isn't always so sparkling. This up attitude is what keeps you so in with higher-ups and the hunk who wants you to join him for a romantic trip to the desert.

"Ultimately, you've learned that no matter how bad a situation seems in the middle of the night," says Flaherty, "you're bound to wake up with a more positive spin." No wonder you bolt out of bed ready to embrace the world.

Below 11 points: Not Enough Attitude

You waste enormous energy conforming to everyone else's expectations. But this pleased-to-please 'tude comes with a price tag. You lose respect by never disagreeing. You lose credibility by constantly apologizing. You lose money because you can't tell the cashier he's rung up an eleven-cent knickknack as eleven dollars! And ultimately, you lose yourself because you won't let on that you have a sense of humor, fresh ideas, and your own devilish desires.

As a child, you might have learned that the only way to be loved was to be agreeable, says Salmansohn. If you became angry, you were probably punished. But wimpy doesn't work in the adult world. If you don't have confidence in your right to happiness, no one else will either.

You *can* end this losing game. For starters, change your posture and tone of voice, and look people in the eye; hunching over and mumbling just doesn't cut it. Directness also counts: "Don't ask someone 'Could you do this?' when 'Would you do this?' is what you really mean," explains Flaherty.

And finally, a little selfishness goes a long way. Do something nice for yourself at least once a day. When you know that you deserve the best life has to offer, the rest of the world will too. ✳

What's Your
Emotional Age **?**

Acting your age can be tricky if you're perma-
nently stuck in a psychological time warp. Determine here whether you're a big baby, forever pre-
teen, or growing old prematurely.

"I still don't know what I want to be when I grow up," complains April
Ward,* a 40-year-old freelance film editor from Los Angeles whose
boot-cut jeans, Kate Spade bag, and trendy layered haircut scream
very early twenties. "Friends my age live in the 'burbs with two cars
and two kids and 401(k) plans. . . . They're grown-ups! I'm like a
teenager." Ward isn't moved to invest in a house, seek a permanent
partner, or even commit to a full-time job. "Most people say, 'This
is life, you have to work, you can't run off to the beach on a
Wednesday afternoon just because it's sunny'—but not me," she
says.

We all know people whose emotional maturity seems out of sync
with their chronological age: the 12-year-old baby-sitter who's as
responsible as any nanny, the elderly woman who whizzes around
town on a purple 3-speed with handlebar streamers, or your darling
ex-boyfriend, who couldn't see how his playing football with his buddies on your birthday and your getting spitting mad were in any way
related.

People idle at a particular emotional age for different reasons,
explains David Klimek, Ph.D., a psychologist in Ann Arbor, Michigan.
Klimek once treated a woman whose parents were so busy achieving that they didn't have time to nurture her. Fiercely independent,
she became the president of her own company at age 27, then married a man whom she had impressed with her self-sufficiency. After
the "I do's," however, she turned into Velcro-wife. "He became the

*Some names have been changed

symbolic dad, and she became the clutching, neglected 2-year-old she was inside," says Klimek. Other childhood traumas, such as illness, divorce, and sibling rivalry, can also arrest or accelerate emotional maturity.

Wherever you pop up on the emotional time line, "It's not inherently good or bad to be either old or young for your age," says Susan Heitler, Ph.D., a clinical psychologist in Denver and author of *The Power of Two: Secrets to a Strong and Loving Marriage* (New Harbinger). Being an emotional child, for instance, means you're impulsive and impatient, which can cause trouble, say, in money matters. But spontaneity, resiliency, and a sense of adventure, also childlike traits, means you're creative and that a party isn't a party until you show up. The real problems arise when your emotional age and the expectations of your chronological age are widely out of sync, says Heitler—if, say, inside you feel like a child and want to mess with Play-Doh all day, but you have a job and kids of your own to tend to.

To figure out whether you're a child, teenager, or adult, take this quiz. Then read how you can grow up, loosen up, and get the most out of your life.

1. **When offered chocolates, you:**
   a. Choose 1 and maybe eat it later.
   b. Take little bites of several, leaving most of them half-eaten.
   c. Dog most of the box in less than 30 seconds, then feel a little sick.

2. **You pay your bills:**
   a. On the same day every month.
   b. When you get around to it.
   c. Sporadically—your credit rating's in a complete shambles.

3. **What's your shopping style?**
   a. Impulsive—you look in your closet and wonder what you were thinking.
   b. You're up on the latest trends, so no pushy salesperson's going to convince you to buy anything you don't want.
   c. You hit the stores mainly when you need something specific.

4. **You run into a friend who's been missing in action. You:**
   a. Let out a whoop and rush to hug her.
   b. Say warmly, "Wow, the last time I saw you was, what, six months ago?"
   c. Wait until she comes over, in case she was avoiding you, then return her greeting with the same enthusiasm she offers.

5. **Your best girlfriend calls, sobbing. She says she thinks her man is stepping out on her. You:**
   a. Calm her and ask exactly what happened to make her suspect he's cheating.
   b. Become outraged—how *could* he?
   c. Insist that, in retaliation, you both slip into your hottest dresses and hit the town for a major drink-and-flirt fest.

6. **A fabulous project at work earns you a big, fat promotion. What's the best part about it to you?**
   a. The rush you get when your boss says you've done a great job.
   b. More money, a better title, and a future so bright, you gotta wear shades.
   c. That you finally can score an office, bail on the Xeroxing, and quit taking orders from your pea-brain higher-up.

7. **You like to make love:**
   a. With dimmed lights, scented candles, and soft, sexy music.
   b. Anytime, anyplace, any position—the more spontaneous, the better.
   c. Furtively. If it's forbidden, it's hotter.

8. **Which of the following best describes your sex style?**
   a. Playful, athletic, energetic.
   b. Coy, intense, full of teasing.
   c. Skillful, sweaty, in sync.

9. **What do you like *least* about sex?**
   a. The mess.
   b. The hassle of dealing with birth control and STD prevention.
   c. The times when you don't have an orgasm—you get really crabby.

10. **If someone close to you died, you'd deal with it by:**
    a. Using gallows humor.
    b. Crying as often as you need to.
    c. Throwing yourself into the funeral arrangements to keep busy.

11. You broke up with your last boyfriend because:
a. He wanted to get too serious too quickly—you just wanted to have fun.
b. He was a slacker—you need someone with a little ambition.
c. You were bored—he wasn't intense or romantic enough for you.

12. How do you feel about shaking your thang at a party?
a. After you've got a few drinks in you, you can be convinced.
b. You're the first one on the dance floor, leading the conga line.
c. No way! You don't like making an utter spectacle of yourself.

13. Friends from out of town descend for a week. How do you deal with the domestic turmoil?
a. What turmoil? You love a perma-party.
b. You can deal as long as you don't actually have to give up your bed.
c. You can't wait for things to return to normal, but you try to be a good hostess.

14. You're at an end-of-summer beach party with good friends when someone suggests skinny-dipping. Which is most like you?
a. "Whoo-hoo! Last one in is a wuss!"
b. "I'll go if everyone else does, but I hope no one notices my lumpy butt."
c. "Er, I don't think so. I'll leave my swimsuit on this time, thank you."

15. Someone tells you a dishy secret and asks you not to spill. You:
a. Tell a few people—but if anyone asks, they didn't hear it from you!
b. Only tell the secret if it will hurt someone else *not* to know.
c. Try your best to keep it in, but sometimes things just slip out.

16. Your friends want to set you up. What do you need to know?
a. What time he's picking you up.
b. Why he's still single.
c. What he does for a living.

Scoring

1. a. adult   b. teenager   c. child
2. a. adult   b. teenager   c. child
3. a. child   b. teenager   c. adult
4. a. child   b. adult   c. teenager
5. a. adult   b. child   c. teenager
6. a. child   b. adult   c. teenager

7. a. adult   b. child   c. teenager
8. a. child   b. teenager   c. adult
9. a. adult   b. teenager   c. child
10. a. teenager   b. child   c. adult
11. a. child   b. adult   c. teenager
12. a. adult   b. child   c. teenager
13. a. child   b. teenager   c. adult
14. a. child   b. teenager   c. adult
15. a. teenager   b. adult   c. child
16. a. child   b. teenager   c. adult

Add up your answers for each category. The category in which you have the most responses is your emotional age. Then read up on your age and learn how to get the most out of who you are.

Child
The upside
You're curious, playful, and adventurous—people love spending time with you because you infuse every situation with a sense of fun. You're so expressive of how you feel (sobbing hysterically at a sad movie, say) that nothing gets you down for too long. Because you are so creative and unself-conscious, you'd make a great actress or teacher. At work, you're the one coming up with the hare-brained ideas with a seed of brilliance.

The downside
You're impulsive and impatient, so playing the stock market or being in charge of the household finances can prove costly. Your biggest beef is that no one lets you do what you want, yet you still want others to take care of you. You can be self-centered, and because of your short attention span, you're not always the best mate. Says Heitler, "When a child gets used to a person, he becomes ordinary, and she wants to go on to the next."

How you can change
Make a point of giving something to others each day without expecting anything in return. "If you can learn to nurture someone

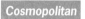

else, then you are on the road to supplanting your self-centered-ness," says Klimek.

Teenager
The upside
You're idealistic, intense, a loyal friend, and will defend your views with passion. Illicit partying with friends is your favorite way to blow off steam. Risk-taking, observant, and intellectually curious, you have a cutting wit that makes people want to be on your good side.

The downside
You can be rebellious, reckless, moody, and noncommittal with plans, and you tend to see the world in black and white. You are often insecure, though you go to lengths to hide it, and are heavily swayed by what your peers think. When office politics divide your workplace, you'll abandon your initial instinct to be on the winning side.

How you can change
Since you have a tough time planning for the long-term future, "try to look at bigger goals," says Klimek. Learn to follow your own instincts rather than automatically reacting to the opinions of others.

Adult
The upside
Secure and confident, you know what you want and how to get it. You take pleasure in achieving at work, and you're a good partner and parent. You're honest with yourself, which allows you to be honest with others.

The downside
You can be too serious, work too hard, feel overwhelmed by responsibilities, and swallow your own needs, which makes you resentful. (Was that *you* exploding at your boyfriend because you sacrificed your gym time to meet him earlier than you wanted?) When you should be having fun—at the movies, with friends, in bed—you get preoccupied with must-dos and forget how to enjoy the moment.

How you can change

"When you feel yourself become tense and say 'Why do *I* always have to do everything?' " says Klimek, "ask yourself, *Is this really the road I want to take?*" Once you're aware that you're doing too much, you can let someone else assume responsibility. ✳

Are You Ambitious or Malicious?

Ask yourself if what you desire and what you must have are the same thing. Unsure? Find out here if you go too far—or not far enough—to get what you want.

1. **It's annual-review time and you want a raise. You would most likely:**
   a. See how you're evaluated before making a move so you don't make waves.
   b. Tell your boss that another company is courting you (whether it's true or not) so you can haggle for a pay increase.
   c. Show her how your responsibilities have grown, then suggest new tasks you'd love to take on.

2. **The grooviest club in town is throwing a record-release bash to which you are not invited. You:**
   a. Phone the club, pretending to work for the label, and get on the list.
   b. Dress to the nines, slip the bouncer fifty dollars, and cruise on in.
   c. Watch all the luminaries go in from behind the velvet ropes.

3. **You feel nauseated in the morning before work, so you:**
   a. Call in sick.
   b. Go in but leave after you discreetly hurl in the ladies' room.
   c. Go in, hurl in the ladies' room, and make sure the boss knows you put in a full day of work anyway.

4. **You suddenly realize that your boyfriend is "the one." You:**
   a. Ask him if he has ever thought about where the relationship is headed.
   b. Drop hints about commitment, children, golden retrievers . . .
   c. Skip your birth-control pill, get pregnant, and pressure him to marry you.

> **Ambition is positive—it's what gets us what we want.**

112

5. **Your job interviewer says he'd like to discuss the position further over cocktails at a hotel. You:**
   a. Politely refuse his obvious maneuver to bring things to a personal level.
   b. Tell him no and immediately withdraw your candidacy.
   c. Go for it! Hey, whatever. A girl's gotta do what a girl's gotta do.

6. **For a big meeting at work, which of the following events would you miss (check any that apply)?**
   a. Your sister's wedding.
   b. A hard-to-get salon appointment.
   c. A nonrefundable cruise you've been planning for the last 6 months.
   d. An unbelievable sale.
   e. The season premiere of your favorite television show.
   f. A dinner at which you are to meet your fiancé's parents.

7. **An apartment in your building just opened up. You want it bad, but so does the woman down the hall. You score the place by:**
   a. Tipping off the landlord to the fact that the other woman has a cat even though the building doesn't allow pets.
   b. Pointing out the many improvements you have made on your own apartment.
   c. Filling out the application and crossing your fingers.

8. **You think about being the boss:**
   a. Every waking minute.
   b. Frequently—it's a matter of making the right strategic moves to get to the top.
   c. Never—who needs all that stress and responsibility?

9. **On weekends, your schedule is:**
   a. Obliterated by all the overflow work you don't have time for during the week.
   b. Completely empty—you sleep and lie around guilt-free, since this is *your* time.
   c. Busy, but filled with stuff you want to do: working out, hanging out with your friends, catching up on reading.

Check each that applies to you:
   10. You've lied on your résumé.
   11. You'd marry a man you don't quite love just for his money or connections.
   12. You only stay at work after hours when you're forced.

13. You would not accept a position that offers a 4-day workweek and long vacations if it were less prestigious than your current job.
14. If offered the answers to a test that would get you a job you want, you'd take them.
15. You would take credit for your assistant's work on your project.

Scoring

1. a–1   b–3   c–2
2. a–3   b–2   c–1
3. a–1   b–2   c–3
4. a–2   b–1   c–3
5. a–2   b–1   c–3
6. a–3   b–1   c–3
   d–1   e–1   f–3
7. a–3   b–2   c–1
8. a–3   b–2   c–1
9. a–3   b–1   c–2

Give yourself the indicated points for each statement you checked:
10. 3   11. 3   12. 0
13. 3   14. 3   15. 3

36 points or more: Ambition Ambush

It's a wonder you found time to take this quiz. Are you surprised to find yourself in this category? Or do you always expect to score the highest, win the title, and be the best no matter what? Well, we have news for you: in this case, getting the highest score means you could be headed for a burnout, baby.

While it's commendable that you work so hard to achieve your goals, it's also scary that you might consider unscrupulous behavior a necessary means to an end. Your brand of all's-fair-in-love-and-war ambition has grown like an out-of-control weed, choking your empathy and making you downright ruthless. "It's wonderful that you don't leave things to chance, but you need to become aware of the little red flags in your life that tell you when you're crossing a line," says Jeanne Segal, Ph.D., author of *Raising Your Emotional Intelligence* (Owl Books). "Maybe you're thirty, and you're already a top executive at a big company, but you also have stomach pains or your back aches or you don't have a meaningful and satisfying relationship."

The good news is, your ambition isn't encoded in your genes. You want to mellow out? "When your eye is on the prize, stop and figure out what moving you in that direction and what you're doing to get it," says Segal. If you're stepping on other people, hurting yourself, or doing unethical things, then you're going too far. You need to find a peaceful balance between what you want and how much of your heart and soul you'll sell to get it.

19 to 35 points: Ambition Ace

Ambition is a drive, and you're at the wheel. Healthy ambition is a skill, a careful balance of self-control, determination, and desire. "A healthy dose of ambition gives us the determination to take risks and get what we want," explains Segal. And your family and friends' definitions of success don't rule you.

You'll work toward a goal despite frustrating obstacles, but you know better than to step on any toes. "You passionately want and need to do something for your own reasons—it's a deep gut feeling," says Segal. Like you, most successful people enjoy the process of achieving as much as reaching their goal.

18 points or fewer: Ambition Anemic

So you're not out to conquer the business world, propel yourself to the top, or marry a millionaire. That's fine . . . if you're where you want to be. But it's hard to believe you don't spend any time imagining a higher-paying job, a nicer house, or a more loving relationship.

A lot of women see ambition as unfeminine or think that success will be at the expense of their family. "Some worry only about the needs of others," says psychologist Joan Steinau Lester, Ph.D., author of *Taking Charge: Every Woman's Action Guide to Personal, Political, and Professional Success* (Conari Press). "Many women need to take themselves more seriously. Ambition is positive—it's what gets us what we want."

So what's stopping you? "You might lack confidence, you might fear failure or feeling vulnerable, but those fears will only derail your

Do's and Don'ts to Getting Ahead

Do: Mention in your interview that you'll work late nights and weekends if that's what it takes to get the job done.

Don't: Elaborate that those late nights and weekends don't have to be limited to the office.

Do: Flirt with that supersexy older tycoon you met at a bar because his power and husband potential turn you on.

Don't: Bring down the government by showing the married-with-children commander-in-chief your flirty, little dental floss G-string.

Do: Speak up with your supersmart suggestions at the monthly ideas' meeting in front of the big cheese.

Don't: Put your cubemate's killer brainstorms in a memo to the big boss and pass them off as your own.

Do: Take your boss to lunch to celebrate her birthday.

Don't: Spend the entire time dishing dirt on your competition for the next promotion.

Do: Be bold and make the first move on that guy you've been eyeing for weeks.

Don't: Put the moves on your best friend's boyfriend when he asks you out for a drink to commiserate about their recent breakup.

Do: Apply for that highly competitive, learn-everything-you'll-ever-need-to-know, once-in-a-lifetime-opportunity internship.

Don't: Tell your handsome young interviewer why Monica's your idol.

goals," says Lester. Convert your fear into productive energy and plan a strategy. Stay the extra hour at work, and let the right people know you've been putting in the extra effort.

Sound like a lot to do? "You can become more ambitious, but you have to expect to do some hard work," continues Lester, who recommends making daily, weekly, and monthly goal lists, always starting with the items that will pay off for *you*. You don't have to be dog-eat-dog at the office or throw all your other responsibilities to the wind, but you do have a personal agenda. "Once you start reaching your goals, you'll feel more satisfied," Lester says.✳

Do: Make your résumé more impressive by focusing on the appealing parts of your experience or making your titles sound more glamorous (i.e., sanitation engineer instead of janitor).

Don't: Claim to have run a company when all you really did was run for coffee.

Do: Arrange a meeting with your boss to tell her why you deserve that big promotion that comes with the corner office.

Don't: Start moving your stuff into the corner office and spreading rumors that you got the gig, just to ward off competition.

Are You a
Giver or a
Grabber?

Do you think it's really much better to receive than to have to give? Are you obsessed with others' needs or just out for yourself? Take this quiz to find out if you're getting—and giving—your fair share.

1. **You and your best friend are invited to a black-tie party. A day before the affair, she has nothing to wear. You:**
   a. Tell her to get her act together and buy something for herself.
   b. Lend her one of your dresses—letting her take the one *you* were planning to wear.
   c. Tell her you'll go shopping with her until she finds the right dress.

2. **Your boss is entertaining clients and invites you to join them for dinner, but your boyfriend is home with the flu and sick as a dog. You:**
   a. Go to the restaurant but ask a friend to bring your boyfriend some soup. You'll skip after-dinner drinks so you can see him as early as possible.
   b. Refuse the invite and spend the entire night nursing your man.
   c. Go to dinner and stay until the delicious end. After all, your boyfriend is a grown man—he should be able to take care of himself just fine.

3. **Your great-aunt dies, leaving you a beautiful antique cabinet. It's just what you could use, but your sister has been coveting it for years. You:**
   a. Keep it, no apologies.
   b. Tell her you'll give her the cabinet if she gives you something to replace it.
   c. Give her the cabinet. You're willing to sacrifice it to make her happy.

4. **You and a coworker both have a pile of work to get through. When she asks you to help her figure out a problem that's hanging her up, you:**
   a. Tell her you can't spare the time.

A "gimme, gimme" attitude can leave you feeling empty.

b. Put your work on hold—even if it means missing *your* deadline—to help her out.

c. Tell her you'll help as long as it doesn't jeopardize your deadline.

5. **When your boyfriend is in the mood for love but you're just in the mood for some sleep, you:**

    a. Suddenly get the proverbial headache and roll over to your side of the bed.

    b. Tell him you're not in the mood, but you'll take a rain check for the morning.

    c. Have sex. You don't want to make him feel hurt or rejected.

6. **You and your roommate are butting heads about who will get the bigger bedroom in your new apartment. How do you deal with the dilemma?**

    a. You let her have her way. You'd rather live with less square footage than tension.

    b. You tell her that if you can't get *your* room, you'll just move.

    c. You work out a compromise; maybe you'll let her have the larger room if you get the extra closet space.

7. **During a romantic dinner, you and your man taste each other's food. The problem: he's salivating over your plate, not his. What do you do?**

    a. Give him a small piece of yours, but eat the rest. You like your meal better too.

    b. Swap plates. You can't stand that look of longing in his eyes.

    c. Scarf down every last bite. Your food is delicious—why should you give any away?

8. **Your mother broke her arm and needs help at home. You:**

    a. Take an unpaid leave and spend your days helping her out.

    b. Go there during your lunch break or after work to see what she needs.

    c. Tell her to hire a helper for the week and then take the opportunity to use her car since she won't be driving it for a while.

9. **You and your girlfriend have the hots for the same man, but he asks you out. What's your next move?**

    a. You go for it. All's fair in love and war.

    b. You ask your friend how she feels about it. If it really bothers her, you'll decline.

    c. You turn him down right away. No man is worth pissing off a friend.

10. Check any statements that apply:

a. When it comes to competitive sports, it isn't about how you play the game; it's whether you win or lose that counts.

b. You're always first to apologize.

c. You'd rather spend Thanksgiving dishing out food in a soup kitchen than pigging out on Mom's home cooking.

d. When you mistakenly receive praise for a colleague's brilliant idea, you make sure she gets the credit.

e. When an elderly woman steps on a crowded bus, you offer her your seat.

f. Even though your man makes less money than you, you always expect him to pick up the tab for dinner.

Scoring

1. a–3 b–1 c–2
2. a–2 b–1 c–3
3. a–3 b–2 c–1
4. a–3 b–1 c–2
5. a–3 b–2 c–1
6. a–1 b–3 c–2
7. a–2 b–1 c–3
8. a–1 b–2 c–3
9. a–3 b–2 c–1
10. Give yourself 3 for a, f; 2 for d, e; 1 for b, c

30 points or more: Grab Hag

There's nothing wrong with going after what you want, but you seem to want it all—all the time. Your "gimme, gimme" attitude probably leaves you feeling empty in the long run. "Grabbers are constantly trying to fill a hole in their soul," asserts Donna Burstyn, a licensed psychotherapist in Beverly Hills, California. "They operate out of fear of not having enough money, enough love, enough attention."

Your must-have-it-all MO could stem from growing up with emotional deprivation, "which can turn into material or emotional greediness," alleges Gail Kalin, a clinical psychologist in the Washington, D.C., area. Or maybe you were poor or had many siblings, so you never had anything that was completely yours. Your selfish behavior could also have developed from the opposite background—growing up as a spoiled only child and feeling entitled to get whatever you want as an adult.

Ironically, the way to fill your emotional hole is to start giving. Burstyn suggests volunteer work as a way to break your grabby habit. Or experiment with small things. Instead of grabbing for something—the last pair of marked-down shoes, the only seat on a bus—let it go and see how it feels. "It might be uncomfortable at first," says Burstyn. "But that means a shift is happening." And after a few stabs at being less selfish, it will start to feel pretty good.

18 to 29 points: Give-and-Take Girl

You definitely understand the joy of giving, but you're generous only when you want to be, not because you feel you have to be. As for getting, you are guilt-free. You can accept gifts and love and friendship because you realize that you deserve all those things. "You probably grew up in a home with an exchange of and respect for one another's ideas," explains Burstyn. And, most likely, your parents were consistently loving and attentive, even when you made mistakes. So your ego was adequately nourished. Think of your give-and-take flexibility as a gift—one that has earned you true friends and healthy relationships.

17 points or fewer: Give-It-All-Away Gal

Generosity is an admirable trait, but really, it's okay to get things too. Your major magnanimity could be a way of overcompensating for not receiving enough parental affection or attention as a child. "Maybe you had to put on a perfect mask for attention," explains Kalin, "so now you feel that you have to buy approval and love."

But acting so altruistically can be like wearing a neon sign that says "Use me!"—and people do. If you're not convinced, Kalin suggests you "write down all the things you've done for someone else in a week, then list what others did for you." If the give list is longer, think about what you gain from your selflessness. Probably not much. In fact, your friends could be so used to getting what they want from you, they might not even know they're taking advantage of you. Try not to be such a pushover. Instead of spending hours listening to your friends' problems, butt in and get some airtime for yourself. Make an after-work date so you have to leave the office rather than stay late to help out a coworker. Once you stop short-changing yourself, you won't lose your friends. Instead, you'll gain their respect and find out just how valuable you are.✳

10 Signs You Give Too Much

1. You're the one everyone calls when they need "a little favor."
2. The last time "no" came out of your mouth, Madonna was still "like a virgin."
3. You're your own little welcome wagon, solely responsible for organizing every office birthday bash, after-work happy hour, and "congrats on your promotion" lunch. Meanwhile, your birthday came and went without a single coworker card and *you* haven't been promoted yet.

4. You'd blow off a date with Matt Damon to bring your sister cough drops.
5. You've yet to see the return of any money lent to former unemployed boyfriends (i.e., every boyfriend you've ever had).
6. The most perfect compliment your man can give you is that you're exactly like his mother.
7. Your friends describe you as a pretty Mother Teresa.
8. You organize your best friend's bachelorette party and wedding shower and spend $400 on her gift, even after she breaks it to you that you're not the maid-of-honor.
9. When you find out your live-in boyfriend's cheating on you, you selflessly tell him you'll stay if he promises not to see her anymore. When he says no, you still agree to neatly pack his things, find him an apartment, and help him move.
10. You hear through the office grapevine that you and your cubemate are up for the same promotion (which you really want). But she's 3 years older and you have time to move ahead, so you make it clear to your boss that she's the better candidate.

What's Your
True Calling ?

Are you destined to be a doctor or a doughnut maker? Do you punch numbers when you really should be delivering punch lines? Take this career quiz to find out how your personality type determines which ladder of success you were born to climb.

1. **You've been invited to a friend's splashy social event. The thing you most look forward to is:**
   a. Meeting new people—like someone special if you are single.
   b. Catching up with old pals.
   c. Putting in a quick, obligatory appearance, then going home.

2. **After a lot of hard work, you've finally reached company-car status, and as a bonus, you even get to choose the model. You pick:**
   a. A showy luxury car with leather seats and a beautiful oak dashboard.
   b. A big 4-wheel-drive Jeep. You want to be able to use the car for off-road camping trips with friends.
   c. Something economical that won't guzzle gas or need a lot of repairs.

3. **You're hosting a large Sunday brunch party. To prepare, you:**
   a. Decorate the invitations, create a festive table setting, and prepare all the food yourself. You get a kick out of organizing events like this.
   b. Call a caterer and have it done professionally. You have much more important things to attend to.
   c. Plan a potluck. That way, everyone gets involved—plus, since you're not cooking, you'll be free to mingle.

4. **Your vacation flight booked 2 months ago has been canceled at the last minute, and the next flight is tomorrow afternoon, making your holiday 1 day shorter. Stuck at the airport, you immediately:**
   a. Take it as an eerie sign and consider postponing the whole trip.

   b. Commiserate with your fellow passengers over the enormous headaches of plane travel, and then settle for what the airline is offering.
   c. Ask to speak directly to a manager and demand that she research your best flight options, even if it means having to take another airline.

> # Do you just *dread* laboring alone or relish working solo?

5. A colleague at work has secured a prestigious position at a different company. Upon hearing the news of her departure, your first instinct is to immediately:

   a. Seize the opportunity to showcase your excellent speech-making skills at her good-bye party in an attempt to wow the corporate bigwigs.
   b. Take her out for a congratulatory farewell lunch and let her know how much she'll be missed.
   c. Calculate how to best compensate workwise for her absence since you know you'll have to take up some slack.

6. You and 2 friends check out that new Italian restaurant that hasn't yet been reviewed. You:

   a. Order a conservative dish like pasta with marinara sauce, assuming they can't possibly screw it up too badly.
   b. Order 3 different entrées for the table and split them all. That way, you get to experiment together, and no one loses out with a dud dish.
   c. Ask the waiter what the best dish in the house is and order that.

7. When going grocery shopping in a supermarket, you:

   a. Visit only the necessary aisles, being careful not to go over the 10-item limit so you can hit the express counter.
   b. Coordinate your shopping list with the store's shelving system. This way, you make a clean trip through the store and avoid revisiting any aisles.
   c. Browse through every aisle. When shopping, you're a slave to your taste buds—plus, you like to check out new products on the market.

8. Embarking on a 6-hour flight on your way to visit relatives, you board the plane to find it half empty. Ecstatic, you:

   a. Take the seat next to the most interesting-looking person you see, with plans of making a new friend.
   b. Seek out an isolated area where you'll be able to spread out and read and relax in peace and quiet.

c. Make a beeline to the stewardess's station and attempt to get bumped up to a barren first-class seat.

9. While relaxing on vacation in the Virgin Islands, the book you choose to read is most likely:
   a. A superemotional love story, like a steamy Danielle Steel novel.
   b. The latest hot biography. You might as well benefit from what you read.
   c. A detective story with lots of descriptive detail and a complicated plotline, like an Ian Fleming novel.

10. A brokenhearted girlfriend calls, bawling about her very recent breakup. You:
   a. Tell her honestly where you think she and her boyfriend went wrong. It's important to advise when you can.
   b. Let her cry on your shoulder. What she needs now is for a trusted friend to be there to listen to her, not lecture her.
   c. Remember when you went through this, and use your experience to come up with ways to make her feel better.

11. After deciding to overhaul your whole apartment, you go shopping for new furniture. Upon entering the first store, you spot the ideal couch. You:
   a. Buy it and have it delivered the very same day, end of story.
   b. Make sure it's a pull-out. You like to invite friends to stay over.
   c. Feel you should look in more stores, in case there's a better pattern you haven't seen or better price.

Scoring

1. a–L   b–S   c–T
2. a–L   b–S   c–T
3. a–T   b–L   c–S
4. a–T   b–S   c–L
5. a–L   b–S   c–T
6. a–T   b–S   c–L
7. a–L   b–T   c–S
8. a–S   b–T   c–L
9. a–S   b–L   c–T
10. a–L   b–S   c–T
11. a–L   b–S   c–T

Mostly L's: Leader

When was the last time you let someone else take the wheel, pick the restaurant, or choose the movie? Too long ago to even remember? Going with the flow is hardly your style. That's because you're most comfortable when you run the show. "Leaders have real take-charge attitudes. They're goal-oriented, driven, and usually the ones with the initiative to get things off the ground," says Kenneth V. Hardy, Ph.D., a psychologist in Syracuse, New York.

You're a born decision-maker. "Leaders are opinionated and able to make up their minds quickly," adds Lisa Rike, a personality trainer in Indianapolis who teaches employees how best to use their personal traits in the workplace. Your pet peeve is people who habitually hem and haw. Consequently, you thrive in jobs like emergency medicine, law enforcement, and politics, where you're counted on to make solid, snap decisions without later obsessing over the choice you've made. You're also a risk-taker, especially when the potential payoff is high. You could trade on Wall Street or negotiate big business deals. However, that doesn't mean the only place you flourish is in a fast-paced profession. "With innately charismatic personalities, leaders are able to use their skills in a variety of areas, from heading up a corporate-takeover team to rallying enthusiasm as a teacher in a classroom," says Carole Hyatt, a career strategist in New York City and author of *Women's New Selling Game* (McGraw Hill).

Always ambitious and in tune with the latest trends, you're not the type to grin and bear anything less than the best. Your professional principles? Delegate whenever possible to hasten productivity, and never pass up a profitable opportunity.

Careers to consider: business executive, salesperson, magazine editor, teacher, image consultant, manager, personal trainer, theater director, doctor, stockbroker, TV producer, politician.

Mostly S's: Socializer

Do you find yourself angling to organize every office birthday party or picnic? Is being liked a bigger priority than conquering the business world? If that's the case, then it's probably your people-pleasing instincts that motivate you most. But that doesn't read *pushover.* You're not one; you're simply highly adept at deciphering the human psyche, which makes you great at getting along with others.

"Socializers are very passionate people," explains Rike. "They're the cheerleaders of the working world." With an instinct for small talk, you're at your best in jobs where you can deal with others, whether it's schmoozing corporate clients or brainstorming at an ad agency. "Socializers are also great negotiators," adds Hardy. "If there's a dispute, a socializer can inevitably get the two sides to compromise."

Always the team player, you enjoy involving everyone from the CEO to the coffee gofer in your projects. To you, establishing a firm social foundation takes precedence over stealing the spotlight any day. You prefer aesthetics over function, and you gauge accomplishment by the appreciation you receive from others. If you were to enter a pageant, you'd be a shoo-in for Miss Congeniality.

Careers to consider: public-relations director, public speaker, disc jockey, family doctor or pediatrician, foreign-relations ambassador, retail salesperson, entertainment editor, TV writer.

Mostly T's: Thinker
You love a challenge. Patient and pragmatic, you relish the chance to roll up your sleeves and immerse yourself in a project. "Thinkers have great analytical skills," says Hardy. "They focus on the most minute details, and their ability to conceptualize ideas easily allows them to anticipate exactly where things might go wrong."

In addition, most thinkers have a bit of a split personality. On the one hand, your matter-of-fact manner means you're consistent and accurate—you rarely act on a whim—making you ideal for jobs that require research and restraint, like accounting and computer programming. On the other hand, you have an insatiable curiosity and the keen ability to look within at your raw emotions for inspiration, which explains why you're drawn to the arts and to science.

But whether you choose a career in photography or forensics, you always do your best work when left alone. Your thoughts are organized (though often your work space isn't), and you love the planning and problem-solving process of any undertaking. When it comes to measuring success, you don't rely on outside praise. To you, the act of achieving is reward enough.

Careers to consider: investigative journalist, illustrator, photographer, musician, computer programmer, architect, travel agent, detective, psychologist, gardener, market researcher, scientist. ✳

Real Women Who Turned Their Passion into a Profession

Theresa Duncan

Once upon a time in a small, fluorescent-lit office in Manhattan, there was a book editor named Theresa Duncan who slaved away over technical tomes on Third World economies and global warming—surfing the Internet during her downtime. A lifelong love of children's storybooks led Duncan to kid-oriented sites and products, but she found that most of them lacked the magical charm that makes children's books special. She knew she could do better—so she did. Today, 29-year-old Duncan is a one-woman fairy-tale factory, creating CD-ROM "interactive adventures" for girls. Her first title, *Chop Suey,* was named 1995's CD-ROM of the Year by *Entertainment Weekly.*

Tarina Tarantino

Since Hollywood's elite discovered her insect-inspired jewelry, everyone's been buzzing about this accessories designer. All it took was a unique vision . . . and convincing her boyfriend to sell his car to finance her first order of crystal hair clips. Now her million-dollar company is creating bejeweled beetles, butterflies, and more for big-screen bigwigs such as Cameron Diaz and Madonna.

Jennifer Palmer

For 7 long years, Jennifer Palmer held secure jobs, most recently as manager of a San Francisco Starbucks. But her real love was throwing parties—fabulous, legendary parties. Her annual cross-dressing party drew 250 guests. And her Valentine's bash and December holiday gala were gotta-be-there blowouts. Now she parties for fun *and* profit as founder of her own company, MarketingEdge SF, producing corporate parties and events.

Are You Psychic?

Are your extrasensory skills supernormal or supernatural? Take this quiz and test your talent for fortune-telling—we predict you'll be glad you did.

The phone rings, and you already know who's calling. You start to worry that someone you know is hurt, and, sure enough, a friend has just had an accident. Are these strange coincidences, or could they be something more? Much of what we assume to be intuition is actually the beginning of our psychic powers in action, claims Hans Holzer, Ph.D., author of *Are You Psychic?* (Avery Publishing Group). "It can be as subtle as a hunch or an uncanny feeling, as blatant as a sudden flash of instantaneous knowledge, a voice, or a vision," Holzer says. But what *is* psychic ability? The most popular theory is that telepathy works like a radio transmission, picking up on other people's brain waves instead of sound waves. Another, more whimsical, idea is that psychic visions are glimpses into a whole other realm, like a fourth dimension or collective consciousness.

Psychic experts insist that we all have a sixth sense—the ability to gain knowledge or information without the use of our traditional 5 senses: taste, touch, smell, hearing, and sight. But some people's psychic ability is more developed than others. How strong is yours? Take *Cosmo*'s third-eye exam to find out if your second sight is already 20/20.

1. **Your first impression of someone usually turns out to be:**
   a. Dead-on. You have a knack for sussing out people's true personalities.
   b. So-so. Occasionally, a coworker you deem untrustworthy pleasantly surprises you, but you're usually pretty perceptive about people's intentions.

c. Completely off. You're constantly getting burned by girlfriends who take from you, then turn on you.

2. **Your lovable but absentminded aunt has lost her keys again. You:**
   a. Find them for her almost instantly. Somehow you always seem to know where missing things are hiding.
   b. Conduct a full-scale, room-by-room search of her home and finally locate them 20 minutes later.
   c. Turn her place upside down hunting for them but come up empty-handed.

3. **Your dreams are usually:**
   a. Vivid and realistic. Some have even turned out to be eerily accurate predictions of things that later happened.
   b. Hazy images or stories that sometimes tip you off to something you didn't realize about yourself.
   c. Too racy to print here.

4. **The last time there was a big office shakedown—a boss left or was fired—your reaction was:**
   a. A knowing look. You could tell something scandalous was going to happen.
   b. Mild surprise. You had a feeling that something was up but thought you were just being paranoid.
   c. Jaw-dropping shock. You had absolutely no clue something big was brewing at the office.

5. **A date suggests bagging the tired old dinner-and-a-movie drill, and joining some friends for a day at the races. You:**
   a. Can't wait to play the ponies—you *always* manage to rake in the big bucks when betting is involved.
   b. Reluctantly agree to go along with the group. When it comes to gambling, you usually just break even.
   c. Tell your man you'll sit this one out—you always go broke when betting is involved, and you're saving up for some slamming knee-high boots.

6. **Of the following 3 movies, the one you'd most like to rent is:**
   a. *Firestarter,* the suspenseful Stephen King chiller with Drew Barrymore as a paranormal child prodigy.
   b. *Flatliners,* the heart-stopping (literally!) thriller costarring Julia Roberts, Kevin Bacon, and William Baldwin that mixes medicine and mysticism.

Extrasensory Aerobics

Regular psychic workouts can help you pump up your mystical muscles. Here, Susan Blackmore, Ph.D., and Adam Hart-Davis, Ph.D., authors of *Test Your Psychic Powers* (Sterling), suggest two ESP exercises to try.

SUIT YOURSELF. Sit on one side of a table, with a friend opposite you. Have the friend shuffle a deck of cards, pick up the top card, and concentrate on its suit. Try to "receive" the image, and guess the card's suit. Repeat with the entire deck. By chance, you should get about 10 correct answers. If you do better, your sixth sense is keener than average.

GET INTO THE SWING OF THINGS. Pendulums are based on 19th-century magic practices and are said to channel psychic ability. Make your own by tying one end of a long piece of string to a small weight, like a ring or stone.

Hold the end of the string between your thumb and forefinger and let the weighted end hang down. Say "Clockwise means yes," and mentally tell the pendulum to swing clockwise. After a few moments, the pendulum will start to turn clockwise. Repeat the procedure in the opposite direction with the words "Counter-clockwise means no."

Now, put a die in a cup and shake it without peeking. Dangle the pendulum over the cup. Watch the direction it swings as you ask, "Did I roll a one?" Do the same for numbers 2 through 6 until you get a yes, then see if you're right. Try this 5 times. If you guess correctly at least 3 times out of 5, you and your pendulum have serious power.

c. *The Wizard of Oz*, the classic musical in which Dorothy, Toto, and friends expose the Wonderful Wizard as a fraud.

7. **Sometimes people get a sense about a location the first time they visit it. It's happened that you:**
   a. Have had hunches about the previous occupants of buildings that have turned out to be absolutely true.
   b. Sometimes get a weird vibe about a place, but nothing concrete.
   c. Have thought, *The Manson ranch? Looks like a lovely place . . .*

8. **The last time you bought a gift for someone, the reaction was:**
   a. "Oh, my God, it's exactly what I wanted! How did you know?"
   b. "Hey, this is really nice. Thank you."
   c. "You shouldn't have. No, I mean you *really* shouldn't have."

9. **How many of the following statements are true? (If you check off 4 or 5 statements as true, give yourself an *a*; give yourself a *b* for 2 or 3; and 0 or 1 equals *c*.)**
   - No one has ever been able to pull off a surprise party for you without your finding out about it beforehand.
   - Frequently, when you've been thinking a lot about a friend or relative you have not seen in a while, she calls.
   - You're a much-in-demand successful matchmaker—you always seem to know which couples will click.

- You have a fleeting thought about someone you don't see often and then you run into that person.
- You frequently get a song in your head and then hear it on the radio shortly after, even if it's not a current hit.

Mostly a's: Sixth Sensational

If you don't already have the words "the Amazing" in front of your name, you should. You're one of the rare few who possesses a psychic force this powerful. Whether or not you were already aware of it, this gift has been helping you sense beyond physical reality and act accordingly. "There are powerfully psychic people who haven't even recognized their abilities," says Brianna Zvonar, a spiritual counselor living in Grand Ledge, Michigan. Could you be one of these supernatural sleuths? Maintaining a detailed journal with any vivid dreams, premonitions, and hunches will help keep you mindful of your second sight—and serve as proof of your intuitive ability if those predictions come true!

Mostly b's: Sixth Sensitive

You have begun to unlock your psychic potential, but there's still plenty of power you have not tapped into yet. All that stands between you and a 900 number that would put Dionne Warwick to shame are a few sessions of mental gymnastics. "Psychicness is just like any other talent, like playing the piano," explains Hans Holzer. "Sure, some people are naturally more gifted than others are, but the more you practice, the sharper your third-eye sight becomes." Check out the box on page 130 for some easy exercises that will help you tone your telepathic skills.

Mostly c's: Sixth Senseless

Your second sight is pretty dim, but don't be discouraged. It's probably just your own skepticism that's holding you back from harnessing your psychic powers. "A skeptical attitude creates anxiety, and that can reduce your psychic ability," says Holzer. Rather than always opting for the purely logical answer to everything, experiment with listening more closely to your intuition—for instance, if you have a hunch about something, go for it and see what happens! And try keeping a log of your dreams. When you're asleep, your skeptical mind is at rest, and psychic messages can get through more easily. ✳

Are You a
Trauma Queen?

Would you concoct a crisis just so you could steal a few more minutes in the spotlight? Take this quiz and find out if you thrive on the thrill of chaos.

1. **The novice waxer at your salon has left behind a hideous memento of her handiwork: an oozing scab mustache on your upper lip. You:**
   a. Claim that you're disfigured for life and demand the termination of this torturous wielder of hot wax.
   b. Apply aloe and ask for a refund.
   c. Blame yourself for trusting a beginner and hope you heal okay.

2. **It's your 6-month anniversary—and only one of you remembered. (Hint: It's not him.) You:**
   a. Don't mention it. He doesn't need to remember every relationship milestone.
   b. Stop taking his calls and change your answering machine's outgoing message to "I'm out looking for a man who won't suffer anniversary amnesia."
   c. Give him a guilt trip but let him off the hook once he's apologized.

3. **Your boss is infamous for firing employees before they've had their morning cup of coffee. Mr. Bigwig says he wants to see you tomorrow at 9 A.M. sharp. You're:**
   a. Cool and calm. There's no point worrying about it all night.
   b. Concerned but collected. You review all your projects in preparation for whatever he might bring up.
   c. Convinced you're canned. At home, you down tequila shots and draft a "you'll rue the day" resignation speech.

4. **You step on the scale. You've gained 10 pounds. Your solution:**
   a. Less chocolate, more time at the gym.
   b. Start a nothing-but-lettuce diet and tell everyone to address you as Moo Cow.
   c. Blame it on premenstrual bloating.

5. **At parties, you've been known to (check all that apply):**
   a. Get so drunk that you need 3 people to help you home.
   b. Flirt to make your boyfriend jealous. (Bonus: The flirtee's attached.)
   c. Overdress—on purpose—so all the other women look comparatively dumpy.
   d. Lie or exaggerate the truth about your job, relationship, status, friends, etc., just to liven things up a bit.
   e. Start stories with "Oh, my God, this was the absolute *worst* day of my *entire* life."

6. **You want to have sex, but your man consistently resists your kisses and caresses. You:**
   a. Demand to know what bimbo is sapping his sexual energy.
   b. Fight back the tears and ask him if he still finds you attractive.
   c. Go to sleep—you aren't going to let one out-of-sync night get to you.

7. **You're finishing up one of the all-time most fabulous first dates. You're closing in for a good-night kiss when you let loose a loud burp. You:**
   a. Shriek like a banshee, run inside, and slam the door in his face.
   b. Shrug and say, "I don't know why burps freak people out so much."
   c. Laugh nervously and hope he, too, sees humor in human nature.

8. **You take your 6-year-old niece to the mall—and quickly lose her in a department store's one-day-sale free-for-all. Your first step is to:**
   a. Get in line to snag a slip dress (75 percent off!). She'll find her way back by the time you reach the register.
   b. Head for the Beanie Babies aisle in the nearest toy store. If she isn't there, notify mall security immediately.
   c. Start hysterically shouting her name.

9. **You frequently pick fights with your lovers just so you can get some hot make-up sex.**
   a. True
   b. False

Scoring

1. a–2   b–1   c–0
2. a–0   b–2   c–1
3. a–0   b–1   c–2
4. a–1   b–2   c–0

5. Give 1 point for each answer
6. a–2   b–1   c–0
7. a–2   b–0   c–1
8. a–0   b–1   c–2
9. True–2 False–0

14 or more points: Scene-Stealing Queen

Whether it's caused by a broken heart or a broken nail, you thrive on the blood-pumping rush of a first-class freak-out. So much so, in fact, that you *intentionally* stir things up. "You're a sensation seeker, someone who not only exaggerates situations but creates problems just because you need the attention," says Nancy K. Schlossberg, Ph.D., coauthor of *Going to Plan B: How You Can Cope, Regroup, and Start Your Life on a New Path* (Fireside Books). However, your traumarama lifestyle may be more draining than entertaining. "You make it hard for people to get close to you, because you demand more energy and empathy than anyone can possibly give," says Eric Dlugokinski, Ph.D., professor of psychiatry and behavioral sciences at the University of Oklahoma. As a child, you probably threw temper tantrums in order to get others to notice you—and stuck with it because it worked. But if you keep stirring up problems just so you can be the star of your own real-life soap opera, even your loved ones will stop tolerating you and start ignoring you. You need to change your self-centered P.O.V. The first step is simple: Ask yourself whether the situation really deserves all the energy you're devoting to it. If it doesn't, merely pausing for composure will help calm you down. But if it really is a big deal, the experts suggest finding another way of releasing your energy: work out, write in a journal, or pummel a pillow. Next, you need to start sharing the limelight—you may find that being a good listener is even more rewarding than constantly being the one at center stage.

8 to 13 points: Ms. Mellow-Dramatic

Sometimes you get caught up in the heat of the moment and your emotions run away from you; but for the most part, you roll with life's punches like a boxing pro. Unlike the trauma queen, who will create a scene just so she can star in it, you would never drum up a drama just to keep things interesting. And, because you're guided by logic and reason, you rarely act impulsively on pure emotion. "When you become upset, you're able to express your feelings in a constructive way," says Dlugokinski. Still, you aren't immune to the occasional uncalled-for fever pitch. During those melodramatic moments, try to take a step back from the immediate situation to examine everything else that's going on in your life. More often than not, you'll realize there's a highly combustible combination of things bothering you—and it just took one teeny trauma to set it off. For example, if you're late on a project at work *and* your cat just died *and* you're mad at your boyfriend, you're more likely to go ballistic when the copier breaks. Fortunately, because you're not known for blowing things out of proportion or provoking problems, there will be no shortage of people willing to help you get a grip when you need it.

Fewer than 8 points: Waiting-in-the-Wings Wallflower

No matter how stressful the situation, nothing gets a rise out of you. Others may envy your ability to shake off every offense, but it *is* possible to be too laid-back. You may go with the flow and accept the status quo just to protect yourself from disappointment or to remain in the background. But until you learn to let loose, others will take advantage of your nonassertive nature and walk all over you. Maybe you grew up in a children-are-seen-and-not-heard household and kept things to yourself so you wouldn't bother your parents or other "too busy" people. Or you may just be shy and afraid of attracting attention and looking like a wacko. "But venting your emotions doesn't automatically mean you're needy or have lost all control," says Dlugokinski. In fact, learning how to express yourself thoughtfully is crucial for becoming a strong, independent woman who is *no one's* doormat. Bonus: venting is healthy. Pent-up stress makes you more vulnerable to numerous illnesses ranging from the common cold to heart disease. So take a cue from the trauma queen and let yourself go to emotional extremes—when it's called for, of course. ✳

Are You Too
Self-Absorbed?

Have you lived on Planet Me so long that you've become an alien to friends? Take this quiz and find out whether you're a prima donna . . . or a pushover.

1. You're walking down the street with your pal, who's been working out like a demon and has dropped 20 pounds (in all the right places), when you notice a lot of male heads turning. You:

a. Assume they're checking you out—it was worth letting your hairdresser take you a few shades lighter.

b. Figure maybe if you hang out with her more often, someone might take a second look at you too.

c. Feel thrilled she's getting the eye.

2. When your 10-year high school reunion comes up, you feel:

a. Worried that no one's going to care what's happened to you in the past decade.

b. Psyched to tell all about your life.

c. Excited to catch up on friends' lives.

3. A coworker is on the phone when you go into her office. You:

a. Stand there until she gets off.

b. Make a motion to give you a buzz as soon as she gets off.

c. Hope you didn't intrude and slink off.

4. Your boyfriend's Wall Street bonus isn't going to be as big as he thought. Your first reaction is to:

a. Tell him you've been wanting to dine at home more often anyway.

b. Worry about whether you'll still get a great Christmas gift.

c. Tiptoe around him and let him vent.

5. **Your friend just caught her husband cheating—with her sister. When she comes to you for some cry time, you:**
   a. Take her out for a stiff martini.
   b. Tell her she can live with you rent-free for as long as she likes.
   c. Say, "Maybe I'd better start keeping a closer eye on *my* sister."

6. **Your company's being taken over. You'll still be on board, but your boss is on her way out. You:**
   a. Think, *Damn—she better put through for my expenses before she gets axed.*
   b. Offer to take her to lunch—be an ear.
   c. Tell her, "The only reason they're keeping me is because I don't cost much."

7. **Right in the middle of your best friend's breaking the news that she's become engaged, you:**
   a. Flag down the waitress and tell her to bring over a bottle of Moët.
   b. Flag down the waitress and tell her to make your shrimp quesadilla extra spicy.
   c. Wonder why you're the first person she's sharing her good news with.

8. **When you go out to buy a friend a gift, your purchase is:**
   a. Something too expensive—but how else can you hold on to her friendship?
   b. Something you'd love to have.
   c. Something she's been talking about—but would never buy for herself.

9. **It's Christmas, and you're going over your flight information with your mom, who's busy cooking dinner for 20. You:**
   a. Opt to splurge and take a taxi home.
   b. Offer to rent a car at the airport and pick up Aunt Harriet on your way.
   c. Remind her what time she has to pick you up from the airport.

10. **Check any of the following statements that apply to you:**
    a. You relish hearing every detail of your girlfriends' love lives.
    b. You realize nobody in your therapy group has any idea about your problems.
    c. "You think you have problems—listen to mine" is a favorite catchphrase.
    d. A week doesn't go by when you haven't been waxed, manicured, plucked, and massaged.
    e. You fix friends up—and make sure they return the favor.
    f. You meet dates at the restaurant—why should they have to spend an extra 20 minutes picking you up at your door?

Scoring
1. a–3   b–1   c–2
2. a–1   b–3   c–2
3. a–3   b–2   c–1
4. a–2   b–3   c–1
5. a–2   b–1   c–3
6. a–3   b–2   c–1
7. a–2   b–3   c–1
8. a–1   b–3   c–2
9. a–2   b–1   c–3
10. Give yourself 3 for c, d; 2 for a, e; 1 for b, f.

24 or more points: Primo Prima Donna

Who cares if the planet were about to go into nuclear meltdown? You'd still be demanding to know why your hairdresser's late for your appointment! Utterly wrapped up in yourself, you're completely unable to see—never mind focus on—others' needs. You push to the front of the movie line, take it as a personal slight if a friend cancels lunch because her dad's in the hospital, steamroll others' crises with a "You think you have it bad?" attitude.

Why the prima donna complex? A self-absorbed person was probably overindulged as a child, says Gail Kalin, a clinical psychologist in Washington, D.C. "Her parents simply may not have had the wherewithal to discipline her," explains Kalin. "So when she goes off into the real world, she has no clue that not everything revolves around her—that other people have needs too." As a result, you never learned the art of empathy—listening to others and understanding what they're going through.

If you've heard the phrase "enough about you" more times than *I Love Lucy* has been on TV, maybe it's time to tune in to others. "Next time someone comes to you with a problem, focus on her feelings first," suggests clinical psychologist Claude Steiner, author of *Achieving Emotional Literacy* (Avon Books). "Say, 'I know how you feel, and I'm sorry you feel so badly.' Ask questions about what she's going through—and bite your tongue when you get the urge to talk about yourself."

Finally, force yourself to come up with ways you can help others—even a stranger, suggests Kalin. "Think of Jack Nicholson in

7 Clues You're Clued in to Others

- Girlfriends call you for man advice.
- Your mom never has to remind you to phone Grandma and Grandpa.
- Your boyfriend has never uttered, "Can you just think about me for once?"
- At restaurants or movies, you're never asked to keep your voice down.
- The boss always taps you for jobs involving people skills.
- You never forget friends' birthdays.
- People don't mind doing you favors.

As Good as It Gets," says Kalin. "He was completely self-absorbed because of his obsessive-compulsive disorder. But his character began to transform when he started taking care of his neighbor's dog. When you do something for someone else, you stop being self-absorbed." So get out there and baby-sit, adopt a pet, volunteer. Isn't it time you joined the *humane* race?

16 to 23 points: Give-and-Taker

The words *But what about me?* rarely enter your head. When people come to you, you genuinely listen to their woes. Still, you're no pushover; you know when others are putting you on overload—and you know how to tell them gently "Enough already." Which is why you've managed to maintain such a wide circle of friends—who rarely find you in a resentful mood.

"You attend to your own needs when life requires it," says Kalin. "Even healthy people become self-absorbed during a personal crisis." Ultimately, a balanced person may choose to make sacrifices for another, "but it's a conscious choice, not a show of martyrdom," says Kalin.

15 or fewer points: Major Martyr

Yes, there's an absorption problem here, but it hardly involves the word "self." If anything, you're a sponge, soaking up everybody else's traumas. But all this giving leaves you no energy to mop up your own spills—in other words, none of this self-sacrifice is getting you anywhere. How did you develop this paper-towel syndrome? "Your parents may not have paid attention to your needs when you were growing up, so as a result, you learned that your needs didn't count," explains Kalin. "Instead, you became incredibly attuned to others' emotions. You felt it was your job to make Mom and Dad happy—and now, you feel you're responsible for every-body else's well-being, even if it's at your own expense."

The thing is, no one's going to want to hang out with a person whose every action screams "Use me!"—except, of course, users. So how do you lose the martyr complex? First off, you have to learn to be your own caretaker. "Every day, write a list of your physical, emotional, intellectual, and spiritual needs," counsels Kalin. Then make time each day to check off at least 3.

Of course, you'll have less trouble getting up the gumption to make demands if you make them sound enticing—or at least fair, suggests Kalin. For instance, tell your man, "I always go to sci-fi movies with you—wouldn't it be fun to try that new comedy?" So next time you feel yourself slipping into don't-worry-about-me mode, pinch yourself—as a reminder that it's not your job alone to fix the planet. ✳

Do You Have a **Healthy Ego?**

Are you your own biggest fan, or is your self-esteem so low, you're convinced you're a major loser?

Part One

1. Your ideal time to hit the gym is:
   a. When it's packed. If you've got it, you may as well flaunt it.
   b. When a friend can go with you, so you don't have to fly solo.
   c. When it's empty. Why should you put yourself on display?
   d. Whenever you can fit it in, preferably when there's no line for a treadmill.

2. When a man passes you on the street and does a total double take, you're convinced:
   a. You're having a *really* good hair day.
   b. He's looking at someone else.
   c. He wants to go to bed with you.
   d. There's something green and leafy stuck between your teeth.

3. At business meetings, you think your opinion is:
   a. Pretty much ignored.
   b. Highly respected.
   c. Appreciated in certain circumstances.
   d. An absolute necessity.

> Give yourself credit—like you would anyone else—when due.

4. You're at an art gallery, checking out a painting that you don't understand. When the artist comes by and starts discussing its symbolism, you:
   a. Tell her it lacks star quality.
   b. Nod your head knowingly, even though you'd probably have an easier time understanding Bantu.

   c. Ask her questions. You're interested in hearing her take on it.
   d. Panic and try to hide your cluelessness with intellectual double-talk.

5. **You have 8 P.M. dinner plans with the man you're seeing. When he's a no-show at 8:30, you:**
   a. Make a move on the guy sitting next to you at the bar and ignore your date when he walks in.
   b. Are shown to your table and order your meal. You're starving!
   c. Assume you've been stood up and head out the door.
   d. Worry you screwed up the plans.

6. **You and an acquaintance get into a heated political debate at a party. As his voice gets louder and an audience starts to gather, you:**
   a. Nearly die of embarrassment, then quickly excuse yourself.
   b. Start agreeing with him, hoping he'll ease up.
   c. Raise your voice a few decibels over his; he's dead wrong.
   d. Stick to your guns and suggest you move to an onlooker-free corner.

7. **A coworker is describing a fabulous Kate Spade bag she bought. You've never heard of the designer, so you:**
   a. Wait for someone else to ask whom they're all talking about, then jump in.
   b. Admit you don't know of her and ask for a more detailed description of the bag.
   c. Figure that she's just another fad, then go on about *your* most recent purchase.
   d. Assume she'll think you're a fashion fool and just keep your mouth shut.

8. **You're at the beach with your beau and decide to take a dip. On your way back, you spot him gabbing with a woman in a barely-there bikini. You:**
   a. Feel like an unwanted whale and dive right back into the water.
   b. Join them in their chat. So what if she looks good; he's with you.
   c. Wait till she takes off; you don't want to interrupt their talk.
   d. Saunter over, making sure your man sees all the men ogling you.

Part Two
Mark each statement true or false:
   1. You'd rather have a cavity filled than get into a confrontation.
   2. Ask a man out? Not in this lifetime.
   3. You'd much rather have sex with the lights turned on than turned off.

4. Karaoke is not in your repertoire.
5. You've asked your boss for a raise.

Scoring
Part One
1. a–4   b–2   c–1   d–3
2. a–3   b–2   c–4   d–1
3. a–1   b–3   c–2   d–4
4. a–4   b–1   c–3   d–2
5. a–4   b–3   c–1   d–2
6. a–1   b–2   c–4   d–3
7. a–2   b–3   c–4   d–1
8. a–1   b–3   c–2   d–4

Part Two
1. T–0   F–2
2. T–0   F–2
3. T–2   F–0
4. T–0   F–2
5. T–2   F–0

35 points or more: Egocentric

You're convinced friends hang on your every word, men live to be with you, and you deserve the corner office. Sure, it's fine to feel good about who you are, but your inflated sense of self could leave you with a fan club of just one.

If you have a need to see yourself as perfect or act as if nothing bothers you, you're probably covering up insecurity, explains Martha Beck, Ph.D., a sociologist in Phoenix and author of *Breaking Point: Why Women Fall Apart and How They Can Re-create Their Lives* (Times Books). "You don't let flaws show for fear you won't be liked." Ironically, Beck says, those "I'm so perfect" signals you send could turn people off, not on.

Try letting your guard down—slowly and carefully. If you consider your looks to be a huge part of your fabulousness, for example, "Go to lunch with a close friend and come clean that you wouldn't be caught dead without makeup," suggests Beck. You'll see that revealing some vulnerability won't push people away—it will only draw them to you.

25 to 34 points: Ego-Stable

Voicing an unpopular point of view, hitting on a man, even admitting you are clueless doesn't faze you. Why? You've fine-tuned your coping skills, which has given you a rock-solid sense of self. Maybe it's because you come from a supersupportive family. Or perhaps you realize that screwing up is a fact of life; everyone does it—and lives to talk about it.

"The key to your confidence is being able to accept yourself—the good and the bad," says Stella Vlamis, a clinical social worker in Staten Island, New York. "You also know that criticism can be constructive. If it isn't, you let it go." If a friend thinks your favorite outfit is a fashion faux pas, you don't rip it up and use it for rags. You think it looks great, which makes you feel great. And that's what really counts.

15 to 24 points: Ego So-So

Fear of going against the flow or making a mistake keeps you in low-profile limbo. And thanks to a high dose of self-doubt, when you dare to tiptoe out on a limb once in a while, you put yourself through the emotional wringer. Maybe you were pushed to perfection by too demanding parents and you still think you need to score a perpetual A+ to be accepted, suggests Beck. Or perhaps you've set your own unattainable standards, which could put a dent in even the most intact self-esteem.

"You need to start trusting your own instincts and not worry so much about what others think," explains Vlamis. "You must have done some things right along the way. Realize those were *your* judgment calls, and they were pretty good."

You can also strengthen your shaky ego by setting new—realistic—goals, suggests Beck. Say you've been keeping your lips locked at work for fear you'll be shot down. Invest in self-esteem security and go to the next meeting armed with ideas. You'll come across as smart and self-assured, which in turn will give you the confidence to strut your stuff again, and again, and. . . You get the idea.

14 points or fewer: Ego-Sorry

You've convinced yourself you're a world-class loser and that the rest of the world would wholeheartedly agree.

"You have to give yourself credit, like you would anyone else, when it's due," says Vlamis. When you and a man mesh or a friend flips over a gift you gave her, tell yourself over and over how great you feel—until you truly believe it. And don't downplay a compliment. Just accept it, think about what's been said, and add it to your credit-worthy repertoire.

Once your confidence level has gone up a few notches, Vlamis says it's time to pry yourself out of the woodwork, but take it one small step at a time. Doing something as insignificant as wearing citrus pants instead of your basic black will push you under a dim limelight—among your friends, who know your style—which will probably feel surprisingly good.

But don't fool yourself. Most seemingly self-assured people suffer from self-doubt. The truth is, everyone has insecurities. The trick is pretending you don't. ✳

Quiz Credits

"Are You a Commitment-Phobe?" by Mary K. Moore

"Are You a Together-Forever Couple?" by John Searles

"Are You Holding Out for a Fantasy Man? (or, Are You Too Willing to Settle?)" by Mary Ganske

"Is He Worthy of Your Love?" by Barrie Gillies

"Do You Sabotage Your Relationships Without Realizing It?" by Dominique DesCordobes

"Can You Trust Him?" by Megan Fitzmorris

"Is He a Keeper?" by Sarah Miller

"What Type of Men Do You Attract?" by Carolyne Bushong

"How Deep Is Your Love?" by Louis Janda (reprinted with permission from author)

"*Cosmo's* Ultimate Couple's Quiz: Are You Combatable or Compatible?" by Barrie Gillies and Lisa Simmons

"How Good Is Your Sexual Etiquette?" by Mary K. Moore

"How Bare Do You Dare?" by Mary K. Moore

"Will Your Sex Life Sizzle Forever or Fizzle Fast?" by Ann Hond

"Are You a Tease?" by Mary K. Moore and John Searles

"What Kind of Sexual Vibe Do You Give Off?" by S. Fever

"How Adventurous Are You in Bed?" by Megan Fitzmorris

"*Cosmo*'s Sexual Aptitude Test" by Megan Fitzmorris

"Are You High Maintenance?" by Rebecca Randolph

"Do You Need an Attitude Adjustment?" by Tamara Weinstein

"What's Your *Emotional* Age?" by Stephanie Dolgoff

"Are You Ambitious or Malicious?" by Jodi Bryson

"Are You a Giver or a Grabber?" by Jane Katz

"What's Your True Calling?" by Jay S. Heflin

"Are You Psychic?" by Robyn Brown

"Are You a Trauma Queen?" by Megan Fitzmorris

"Are You Too Self-Absorbed?" by Barrie Gillies and Lisa Simmons

"Do You Have a Healthy Ego?" by Amy M. Nebens

Additional writing by Karina Vaysburd